Guidelines for
the treatment of malaria

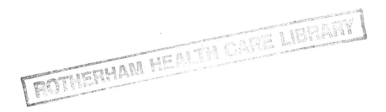
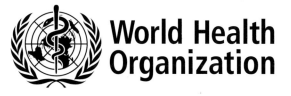

**World Health
Organization**

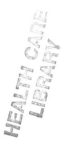

WHO Library Cataloguing-in-Publication Data

Guidelines for the treatment of malaria/World Health Organization.

Running title: WHO guidelines for the treatment of malaria.

1. Malaria – drug therapy. 2. Malaria – diagnosis. 3. Antimalarials – administration and dosage. 4. Drug therapy, Combination. 5. Guidelines. I. Title. II. Title: WHO guidelines for the treatment of malaria.

ISBN 92 4 154694 8   (NLM classification: WC 770)
ISBN 978 92 4 154694 2   WHO/HTM/MAL/2006.1108

For technical information, please contact:

Dr P. Olumese

Global Malaria Programme
World Health Organization
20, avenue Appia – CH-1211 Geneva 27
Tel. +41 22 791 4424
Fax +41 22 791 4824
E-mail: olumesep@who.int

Printed in Switzerland
Design: B. Duret – Cover: T. Cailler

18439

Contents

GLOSSARY

Artemisinin-based combination therapy (ACT). A combination of artemisinin or one if its derivatives with an antimalarial or antimalarials of a different class.

Asexual cycle. The life-cycle of the malaria parasite in host red blood cells (intra-erythrocytic development) from merozoite invasion to schizont rupture (merozoite → ring stage → trophozoite → schizont → merozoites). Duration approximately 48 h in *Plasmodium falciparum*, *P. ovale* and *P. vivax*; 72 h in *P. malariae*.

Asexual parasitaemia. The presence in host red blood cells of asexual parasites. The level of asexual parasitaemia can be expressed in several different ways: the percentage of infected red blood cells, the number of infected cells per unit volume of blood, the number of parasites seen in one microscopic field in a high-power examination of a thick blood film, or the number of parasites seen per 200–1000 white blood cells in a high-power examination of a thick blood film.

Cerebral malaria. Severe falciparum malaria with coma (Glasgow coma scale <11, Blantyre coma scale <3). Malaria with coma persisting for >30 min after a seizure is considered to be cerebral malaria.

Combination treatment (CT). A combination of two or more different classes of antimalarial medicines with unrelated mechanisms of action.

Cure. Elimination of the symptoms and asexual blood stages of the malaria parasite that caused the patient or carer to seek treatment.

Drug resistance. Reduced susceptibility of the causal agent to a drug. WHO defines resistance to antimalarials as the ability of a parasite strain to survive and/or multiply despite the administration and absorption of a medicine given in doses equal to – or higher than – those usually recommended but within the tolerance of the subject, with the caveat that the form of the drug active against the parasite must be able to gain access to the parasite or the infected red blood cell for the duration of the time necessary for its normal action. Resistance to antimalarials arises because of the selection of parasites with genetic mutations or gene amplifications that confer reduced susceptibility.

Gametocytes. Sexual stages of malaria parasites present in the host red blood cells, which are infective to the anopheline mosquito.

Hypnozoites. Persistent liver stages of *P. vivax* and *P. ovale* malaria that remain dormant in host hepatocytes for a fixed interval (3–45 weeks) before maturing to hepatic schizonts. These then burst and release merozoites, which infect red blood cells. Hypnozoites are the source of relapses.

Malaria pigment (haemozoin). A dark brown granular pigment formed by malaria parasites as a by-product of haemoglobin catabolism. The pigment is evident in mature trophozoites and schizonts.

Merozoites. Parasites released into the host bloodstream when a hepatic or erythrocytic schizont bursts. These then invade the red blood cells.

Monotherapy. Antimalarial treatment with a single medicine (either a single active compound or a synergistic combination of two compounds with related mechanism of action).

Plasmodium. A genus of protozoan vertebrate blood parasites that includes the causal agents of malaria. *Plasmodium falciparum*, *P. malariae*, *P. ovale* and *P. vivax* cause malaria in humans.

Pre-erythrocytic development. The life-cycle of the malaria parasite when it first enters the host. Following inoculation into a human by the female anopheline mosquito, sporozoites invade parenchyma cells in the host liver and multiply within the hepatocytes for 5–12 days, forming hepatic schizonts. These then burst liberating merozoites into the bloodstream, which subsequently invade red blood cells.

Radical cure. In *P. vivax* and *P. ovale* infections only, this comprises cure as defined above plus prevention of relapses.

Rapid diagnostic test (RDT). An antigen-based stick, cassette or card test for malaria in which a coloured line indicates that plasmodial antigens have been detected.

Recrudescence. The recurrence of asexual parasitaemia after treatment of the infection with the same infection that caused the original illness (in endemic areas now defined by molecular genotyping). This results from incomplete clearance of parasitaemia by treatment and is therefore different to a relapse in *P. vivax* and *P. ovale* infections.

Recurrence. The recurrence of asexual parasitaemia following treatment. This can be caused by a recrudescence, a relapse (in *P. vivax* and *P. ovale* infections only) or a new infection.

Relapse. The recurrence of asexual parasitaemia in *P. vivax* and *P. ovale* malaria deriving from persisting liver stages. Relapse occurs when the blood stage infection has been eliminated but hypnozoites persist in the liver and mature to form hepatic schizonts. After a variable interval of weeks (tropical strains) or months (temperate strains) the hepatic schizonts burst and liberate merozoites into the bloodstream.

Ring stage. Young usually ring-shaped intra-erythrocytic malaria parasites, before malaria pigment is evident under microscopy.

Schizonts. Mature malaria parasites in host liver cells (hepatic schizonts) or red blood cells (erythrocytic schizonts) that are undergoing nuclear division. This process is called schizogony.

Selection pressure. Resistance to antimalarials emerges and spreads because of the selective survival advantage that resistant parasites have in the presence of antimalarials that they are resistant to. Selection pressure describes the intensity and magnitude of the selection process; the greater the proportion of parasites in a given parasite population exposed to concentrations of an antimalarial that allow proliferation of resistant, but not sensitive parasites, the greater is the selection pressure.

Severe anaemia. Haemoglobin concentration of <5 g/100 ml.

Severe falciparum malaria. Acute falciparum malaria with signs of severity and/or evidence of vital organ dysfunction.

Sporozoites. Motile malaria parasites that are infective to humans, inoculated by a feeding female anopheline mosquito. The sporozoites invade hepatocytes.

Transmission intensity. The intensity of malaria transmission measured by the frequency with which people living in an area are bitten by anopheline mosquitoes carrying sporozoites. This is often expressed as the annual entomological inoculation rate (EIR), which is the number of inoculations of malaria parasites received by one person in one year.

Trophozoites. Stage of development of the malaria parasites within host red blood cells from the ring stage and before nuclear division. Mature trophozoites contain visible malaria pigment.

Uncomplicated malaria. Symptomatic infection with malaria parasitaemia without signs of severity and/or evidence of vital organ dysfunction.

ABBREVIATIONS

ACT	artemisinin-based combination therapy
AL	artemether-lumefantrine combination
AQ	amodiaquine
AS	artesunate
AS+AQ	artesunate + amodiaquine combination
AS+MQ	artesunate + mefloquine combination
AS+SP	artesunate + sulfadoxine-pyrimethamine combination
CI	confidence interval
CQ	chloroquine
EIR	entomological inoculation rate
HIV/AIDS	human immunodeficiency virus/ acquired immunodeficiency syndrome
HRP2	histidine-rich protein 2
IC_{50}	concentration providing 50% inhibition
MIC	minimum inhibitory concentration
MQ	mefloquine
OR	odds ratio
PCR	polymerase chain reaction
*p*LDH	*parasite*-lactate dehydrogenase
RCT	randomized controlled trial
RDT	rapid diagnostic test
RR	relative risk
SP	sulfadoxine–pyrimethamine
WHO	World Health Organization
WMD	weighted mean difference

1. INTRODUCTION

1.1 Background

Malaria is an important cause of death and illness in children and adults in tropical countries. Mortality, currently estimated at over a million people per year, has risen in recent years, probably due to increasing resistance to antimalarial medicines. Malaria control requires an integrated approach comprising prevention including vector control and treatment with effective antimalarials. The affordable and widely available antimalarial chloroquine that was in the past a mainstay of malaria control is now ineffective in most falciparum malaria endemic areas, and resistance to sulfadoxine–pyrimethamine is increasing rapidly. The discovery and development of the artemisinin derivatives in China, and their evaluation in South-East Asia and other regions, have provided a new class of highly effective antimalarials, and have already transformed the chemotherapy of malaria in South-East Asia. Artemisinin-based combination therapies (ACTs) are now generally considered as the best current treatment for uncomplicated falciparum malaria.

These treatment guidelines recommend antimalarials for which there is adequate evidence of efficacy and safety now, and which are unlikely to be affected by resistance in the near future. Much of the world's symptomatic malaria is treated in peripheral health centres or remote villages, where facilities are limited. The aim is therefore to provide simple and straightforward treatment recommendations based on sound evidence that can be applied effectively in most settings.

These guidelines are based on a review of current evidence and are developed in accordance with WHO's standard methodology. Clinical evidence has been assessed in an objective way using standard methods. The number of anti-malarial drug trials published has doubled in the past seven years, so these guidelines have a firmer evidence base than previous treatment recommen-dations. Inevitably, information gaps remain, however, and so the guidelines will remain under regular review and will be updated as new evidence becomes available. There are also difficulties when comparing results from different areas, as levels of drug resistance and background immunity vary. Where transmission levels and, consequently, immunity are high, the malaria symptoms are self-limiting in many patients, in particular in adults, so that drugs that are only partially effective may appear still to work well in many cases, misleading patients and doctors alike. But in the same location, the young child who lacks immunity to illness caused by P. falciparum may die if ineffective drugs are given.

The treatment recommendations given in these guidelines aim for effective treatment for the most vulnerable and therefore take all the relevant factors into account. These factors include laboratory measures, such as tests for *in vitro* antimalarial susceptibility and validated molecular markers of resistance, the pharmacokinetic and pharmacodynamic properties of the different antimalarials, and clinical trial results. Cost is a factor that has been taken into consideration in antimalarial treatment policy and practices. However, there are increasing international subsidies for antimalarials. Efficacy (both now and in the future) and safety have therefore taken precedence when making the recommendations. The malaria treatment guidelines given below are brief; for those who wish to study the evidence base in more detail, a series of annexes is provided.

1.2 Objectives and target audience

1.2.1 Objectives

The purpose of this document is to provide comprehensible, global, evidence-based guidelines to help formulate policies and protocols for the treatment of malaria. Information is presented on the treatment of:

- uncomplicated malaria, including disease in special groups (young children, pregnant women, people who are HIV-positive, travellers from non-malaria endemic regions) and in epidemics and complex emergency situations;
- severe malaria.

The guidelines do not deal with preventive uses of antimalarials, such as intermittent preventive treatment or chemoprophylaxis.

1.2.2 Target audience

The guidelines are aimed primarily at policy-makers in ministries of health. The following groups should also find them useful:

- public health and policy specialists working in hospitals, ministries, non-governmental organizations and primary health care services;
- health professionals (doctors, nurses and paramedical officers).

The guidelines provide a framework for the development of specific and more detailed treatment protocols that take into account national and local malaria drug resistance patterns and health service capacity (see Annex 2). They are not intended to provide a comprehensive clinical management guide for the treatment of malaria. However, where there are controversies about specific clinical practices, and evidence is currently available to provide information to guide decision-making about these practices, that information has been included.

1.3   Methods used in developing the guidelines and recommendations

These guidelines have been developed in accordance with the *WHO Guidelines for Guidelines Development*.[1] In order to ensure that the guidelines are based on the best current evidence, WHO commissioned two academic centres to identify, compile and critically review published and unpublished studies of antimalarial treatments. The collated evidence was then reviewed by the Technical Guidelines Development Group made up of a broad spectrum of experts on malaria, malaria control programmes, and treatment guidelines methodology. A large number of external reviewers with a wide range of expertise were also involved in developing the guidelines.

1.3.1   Evidence considered

In assessing the available information on treatment options, four main types of information were considered, and should also be considered by countries seeking to adapt the guidelines.[2] Wherever possible, systematic reviews of randomized trials that directly compare two or more treatment alternatives in large populations were identified and used as the basis for recommendations. It is clear that such evidence does not exist for all options, but recommendations on these options still need to be made. Other information including studies measuring cure rates but not directly comparing treatments, pharmacological assessments and surveillance data about resistance patterns have therefore also been considered.

In relation to malaria, as with other diseases, systematic reviews are not the sole basis for decision-making: the large differences in transmission intensity, and thus baseline immunity, in treatment populations and in resistance patterns all have major effects on treatment responses. Any statistical analysis that combines the results of individual studies has to take due account of these factors and be interpreted accordingly. However, such analyses do not obviate the need for a systematic and comprehensive review of all available trials before reaching decisions about treatment recommendations.

Treatments for malaria, like those for many infectious diseases, must be considered from the perspective of community or public health benefits and harms as well as from that of the patient. In some instances, therefore, the recommendations provided here are based on public health considerations as well as the potential individual benefits.

---

[1] The process is described in detail in Annex 1.

[2] A guide to assist country adaptation of these guidelines is provided in Annex 2.

Cost-effectiveness studies have not been included in the information considered by the Technical Guidelines Development Group at this stage for two reasons: there are very few completed, generalizable cost-effectiveness studies that relate to the main treatment options being considered and the price of the antimalarials concerned is extremely fluid, rendering such studies unreliable. However, as relevant information becomes available, it will be considered for inclusion in future editions of the guidelines.

1.3.2　Presentation of evidence

For clarity, these guidelines have adopted a simple descriptive approach; this may be revised in future editions. They are presented as a central unreferenced main document containing the recommendations. Summaries of the recommendations are given in boxes. Symbols for the evidence used as the basis of each recommendation (in order of level of evidence) are:

S formal systematic reviews, such as a Cochrane Review, including more than one randomized controlled trial;

T comparative trials without formal systematic review;

O observational studies (e.g. surveillance or pharmacological data);

E expert opinion/consensus.

In addition, for each policy or treatment question leading to a recommendation, a brief summary of evidence is provided in a separate evidence box. Full reviews of the evidence and references are provided in annexes. If pharmacokinetics studies have been included as part of the deliberations, this is noted in the main document.[3]

---

[3] Details of the pharmacology of antimalarials are provided in Annex 3.

2. THE CLINICAL DISEASE

Malaria is caused by infection of red blood cells with protozoan parasites of the genus *Plasmodium*. The parasites are inoculated into the human host by a feeding female anopheline mosquito. The four *Plasmodium* species that infect humans are *P. falciparum*, *P. vivax*, *P. ovale* and *P. malariae*. Occasional infections with monkey malaria parasites, such as *P. knowlesi,* also occur.

The first symptoms of malaria are nonspecific and similar to the symptoms of a minor systemic viral illness. They comprise: headache, lassitude, fatigue, abdominal discomfort and muscle and joint aches, followed by fever, chills, perspiration, anorexia, vomiting and worsening malaise. This is the typical picture of uncomplicated malaria. Residents of endemic areas are often familiar with this combination of symptoms, and frequently self-diagnose.

Malaria is therefore frequently overdiagnosed on the basis of symptoms alone. Infection with *P. vivax* and *P. ovale*, more than with other species, can be associated with well-defined malarial paroxysms, in which fever spikes, chills and rigors occur at regular intervals. At this stage, with no evidence of vital organ dysfunction, the case-fatality rate is low (circa 0.1% for *P. falciparum* infections – the other human malarias are rarely fatal) provided prompt and effective treatment is given. But if ineffective drugs are given or treatment is delayed in falciparum malaria, the parasite burden continues to increase and severe malaria may ensue. A patient may progress from having minor symptoms to having severe disease within a few hours. This usually manifests with one or more of the following: coma (cerebral malaria), metabolic acidosis, severe anaemia, hypoglycaemia and, in adults, acute renal failure or acute pulmonary oedema. By this stage, mortality in people receiving treatment has risen to 15–20%. If untreated, severe malaria is almost always fatal.

The nature of the clinical disease depends very much on the pattern and intensity of malaria transmission in the area of residence, which determines the degree of protective immunity acquired and, in turn, the clinical disease profile. Where malaria transmission is "stable" – meaning where populations are continuously exposed to a fairly constant rate of malarial inoculations – and if the inoculation rates are high – entomological inoculation rate (EIR) >10/year –, then partial immunity to the clinical disease and to its severe manifestations is acquired early in childhood. In such situations, which prevail in much of sub-Saharan Africa and parts of Oceania, the acute clinical disease described above is almost always confined to young children who suffer high parasite densities and acute clinical disease. If untreated, this can progress very rapidly to severe malaria. In stable and high-transmission areas, adolescents and adults are partially immune and rarely suffer clinical disease, although they continue to harbour low blood-parasite densities. Immunity is reduced in pregnancy, and can be lost when individuals move out of the transmission zone.

In areas of unstable malaria, the situation prevailing in much of Asia and Latin America and the remaining parts of the world where malaria is endemic, the rates of inoculation fluctuate greatly over seasons and years. EIRs are usually <5/year and often <1/year. This retards the acquisition of immunity and results in people of all ages, adults and children alike, suffering acute clinical malaria, with a high risk of progression to severe malaria if untreated. Epidemics may occur in areas of unstable malaria when inoculation rates increase rapidly. Epidemics manifest as a very high incidence of malaria in all age groups and can overwhelm health services. Severe malaria is common if effective treatment is not made widely available.

Thus in areas of high transmission, it is children who are at risk of severe malaria and death, whereas in areas of low or unstable transmission, all age groups are at risk.

3. TREATMENT OBJECTIVES

3.1   Uncomplicated malaria

The objective of treating uncomplicated malaria is to cure the infection. This is important as it will help prevent progression to severe disease and prevent additional morbidity associated with treatment failure. Cure of the infection means eradication from the body of the infection that caused the illness. In treatment evaluations in all settings, emerging evidence indicates that it is necessary to follow patients for long enough to document cure (see section 6.1). In assessing drug efficacy in high-transmission settings, temporary suppression of infection for 14 days is not considered sufficient by the group.

The public health goal of treatment is to reduce transmission of the infection to others, i.e. to reduce the infectious reservoir.[4]

A secondary but equally important objective of treatment is to prevent the emergence and spread of resistance to antimalarials. Tolerability, the adverse effect profile and the speed of therapeutic response are also important considerations.

3.2   Severe malaria

The primary objective of antimalarial treatment in severe malaria is to prevent death. Prevention of recrudescence and avoidance of minor adverse effects are secondary. In treating cerebral malaria, prevention of neurological deficit is also an important objective. In the treatment of severe malaria in pregnancy, saving the life of the mother is the primary objective.

---

[4] Further information on antimalarials and malaria transmission is provided in Annex 4.

4. DIAGNOSIS OF MALARIA

Prompt and accurate diagnosis of malaria is part of effective disease manage-ment and will, if implemented effectively, help to reduce unnecessary use of antimalarials.[5] High sensitivity of malaria diagnosis is important in all settings, in particular for the most vulnerable population groups, such as young children, in which the disease can be rapidly fatal. High specificity can reduce unnecessary treatment with antimalarials and improve differential diagnosis of febrile illness.

The diagnosis of malaria is based on clinical criteria (clinical diagnosis) supplemented by the detection of parasites in the blood (parasitological or confirmatory diagnosis). Clinical diagnosis alone has very low specificity and in many areas parasitological diagnosis is not currently available. The decision to provide antimalarial treatment in these settings must be based on the prior probability of the illness being malaria. One needs to weigh the risk of withholding antimalarial treatment from a patient with malaria against the risk associated with antimalarial treatment when given to a patient who does not have malaria.

4.1　Clinical diagnosis

The signs and symptoms of malaria are nonspecific. Malaria is clinically diagnosed mostly on the basis of fever or history of fever. The following WHO recommendations are still considered valid for clinical diagnosis.[6]

- In general, in settings where the risk of malaria is low, clinical diagnosis of uncomplicated malaria should be based on the degree of exposure to malaria and a history of fever in the previous 3 days with no features of other severe diseases.

- In settings where the risk of malaria is high, clinical diagnosis should be based on a history of fever in the previous 24 h and/or the presence of anaemia, for which pallor of the palms appears to be the most reliable sign in young children.

The WHO/UNICEF strategy for Integrated Management of Childhood Illness (IMCI)[7] has also developed practical algorithms for management of the sick child presenting with fever where there are no facilities for laboratory diagnosis.

---

[5]　Further information on the diagnosis of malaria is provided in Annex 5.

[6]　WHO Expert Committee on Malaria. Twentieth report. Geneva, World Health Organization, 2000 (WHO Technical Report Series, No. 892).

[7]　IMCI information package, 1999. Geneva, World Health Organization, 1999 (document WHO/CHS/CAH/98.1).

4.2   Parasitological diagnosis

The introduction of ACTs has increased the urgency of improving the specificity of malaria diagnosis. The relatively high cost of these drugs makes waste through unnecessary treatment of patients without parasitaemia unsustainable. In addition to cost savings, parasitological diagnosis has the following advantages:

- improved patient care in parasite-positive patients owing to greater certainty that the patient has malaria;
- identification of parasite-negative patients in whom another diagnosis must be sought;
- prevention of unnecessary exposure to antimalarials, thereby reducing side-effects, drug interactions and selection pressure;
- improved health information;
- confirmation of treatment failures.

The two methods in use for parasitological diagnosis are light microscopy and rapid diagnostic tests (RDTs). Light microscopy has the advantage of low cost and high sensitivity and specificity when used by well-trained staff. RDTs for detection of parasite antigen are generally more expensive, but the prices of some of these products have recently decreased to an extent that makes their deployment cost-effective in some settings. Their sensitivity and specificity are variable, and their vulnerability to high temperatures and humidity is an important constraint. Despite these concerns, RDTs make it possible to expand the use of confirmatory diagnosis. Deployment of these tests, as with microscopy, must be accompanied by quality assurance. Practical experience and operational evidence from large-scale implementation are limited and, therefore, their introduction should be carefully monitored and evaluated.

The results of parasitological diagnosis should be available within a short time (less than 2 h) of the patient presenting. If this is not possible, the patient must be treated on the basis of a clinical diagnosis.

4.2.1   The choice between RDTs and microscopy

The choice between RDTs and microscopy depends on local circumstances, including the skills available, the usefulness of microscopy for other diseases found in the area, and the case-load. Where the case-load of fever patients is high, microscopy is likely to be less expensive than RDTs. Microscopy has further advantages in that it can be used for speciation and quantification of parasites, and identification of other causes of fever. However, most malaria patients are treated outside the health services, for example, in the community, in the home or by private providers; microscopy is generally not feasible in such circumstances, but RDTs may be.

The following conclusions and recommendations are based on evidence summarized by recent WHO consultations, especially the Technical Consultation on the Role of Parasitological Diagnosis in Malaria Case Management in Areas of High Transmission, held in Geneva from 25 to 26 October 2004 (report in preparation).

4.3 Where malaria transmission is low to moderate and/or unstable

Parasitological confirmation of the diagnosis of malaria is recommended. This should be provided by microscopy or, where not available, RDTs. Low to moderate transmission settings[8] include many urban areas in Africa, and the low transmission season in areas with seasonal malaria.

In settings where malaria incidence is very low, parasitological diagnosis for all fever cases may lead to considerable expenditure to detect only a few patients who are actually suffering from malaria. In such settings, health workers should be trained to identify, through the history, patients that have been exposed to malaria risk before they conduct a parasitological test.

4.4 In stable high-transmission settings

Malaria is usually the most common cause of fever in children under 5 years of age in these areas. Antimalarial treatment should therefore be given to children with fever (>37.5 °C) or a history of fever and no other obvious cause. Malaria is the most likely cause of their illness and there is as yet no evidence to show that the benefits of parasitological diagnosis in this highly vulnerable group outweigh the risks of not treating false negatives. In children of 5 years of age and above, malaria becomes progressively less likely as a cause of fever, as immunity is acquired. In these older children and in adults, malaria diagnosis should be based on a parasitological confirmation. Parasitological diagnosis should be promoted in pregnant women, to improve the differential diagnosis of fever and to reduce unnecessary use of antimalarials in pregnancy. Parasitological diagnosis is also particularly important in settings with a high prevalence of HIV/AIDS because of the high incidence of febrile disease that is not malaria in HIV-infected patients.

---

[8] Transmission intensity is conventionally expressed in terms of EIR (see section 2). There is as yet no consensus on criteria for determining the thresholds between high, and low to moderate transmission settings. Suggested criteria include: the proportion of all children under 5 years of age with patent parasitaemia, and the incidence of individuals with the spleen palpable below the umbilicus in children aged 2–9 years. The IMCI guidelines recommend that areas in which fewer than 5% of young children with fever have malaria parasitaemia should be considered as low-transmission settings.

4.5   Malaria parasite species identification

In areas where two or more species of malaria parasites are common, only a parasitological method will permit a species diagnosis. Where mono-infection with *P. vivax* is common and microscopy is not available, it is recommended that a combination RDT which contains a pan-malarial antigen is used. Alternatively, RDTs specific for falciparum malaria may be used, and treatment for vivax malaria given only to cases with a negative test result but a high clinical suspicion of malaria. Where *P. vivax, P.malariae* or *P.ovale* occur almost always as a co-infection with *P.* falciparum, an RDT detecting *P. falciparum* alone is sufficient. Anti-relapse treatment with primaquine should only be given to cases with confirmed diagnosis of vivax malaria.

4.6   In epidemics and complex emergencies

In epidemic and complex emergency situations, facilities for parasitological diagnosis may be unavailable or inadequate to cope with the case-load. In such circumstances, it is impractical and unnecessary to demonstrate parasites before treatment in all cases of fever. However, there is a role for parasitological diagnosis even in these situations (see section 11.1).

Summary of recommendations on parasitological diagnosis

RECOMMENDATIONS	LEVEL OF EVIDENCE
In areas of low to moderate transmission, prompt parasitological confirmation of the diagnosis is recommended before treatment is started. This should be achieved through microscopy or, where not available, RDTs.	E
In areas of high stable malaria transmission, the prior probability of fever in a child being caused by malaria is high. Children under 5 years of age should therefore be treated on the basis of a clinical diagnosis of malaria. In older children and adults including in pregnant women, a parasitological diagnosis is recommended before treatment is started.	E
In all suspected cases of severe malaria, a parasitological confirmation of the diagnosis of malaria is recommended. In the absence of or a delay in obtaining parasitological diagnosis, patients should be treated for severe malaria on clinical grounds.	E

5. RESISTANCE TO ANTIMALARIAL MEDICINES[9]

Resistance has arisen to all classes of antimalarials except, as yet, to the artemisinin derivatives. This has increased the global malaria burden and is a major threat to malaria control. Widespread and indiscriminate use of antimalarials places a strong selective pressure on malaria parasites to develop high levels of resistance. Resistance can be prevented, or its onset slowed considerably, by combining antimalarials with different mechanisms of action and ensuring very high cure rates through full adherence to correct dose regimens.

5.1   Impact of resistance

Initially, at low levels of resistance and with a low prevalence of malaria, the impact of resistance to antimalarials is insidious. The initial symptoms of the infection resolve and the patient appears to be better for some weeks. When symptoms recur, usually more than two weeks later, anaemia may have worsened and there is a greater probability of carrying gametocytes (which in turn carry the resistance genes) and transmitting malaria. However, the patient and the treatment provider may interpret this as a newly acquired infection. At this stage, unless clinical drug trials are conducted, resistance may go unrecognized. As resistance worsens the interval between primary infection and recrudescence shortens, until eventually symptoms fail to resolve following treatment. At this stage, malaria incidence may rise in low-transmission settings and mortality is likely to rise in all settings.

5.2   Global distribution of resistance

Resistance to antimalarials has been documented for *P. falciparum, P. vivax* and, recently, *P. malariae.*

In *P. falciparum*, resistance has been observed to almost all currently used antimalarials (amodiaquine, chloroquine, mefloquine, quinine and sulfadoxine–pyrimethamine) except for artemisinin and its derivatives. The geographical distributions and rates of spread have varied considerably.

P. vivax has developed resistance rapidly to sulfadoxine–pyrimethamine in many areas. Chloroquine resistance is confined largely to Indonesia, East Timor, Papua New Guinea and other parts of Oceania. There are also documented reports

---

[9] Further information on the emergence, spread and prevention of resistance to antimalarials is provided in Annex 6.

from Peru. *P. vivax* remains sensitive to chloroquine in South-East Asia, the Indian subcontinent, the Korean peninsula, the Middle East, north-east Africa, and most of South and Central America.

5.3   Assessing resistance

The following methods are available for assessing resistance to antimalarials:

- *in vivo* assessment of therapeutic efficacy (see section 6.1),
- *in vitro* studies of parasite susceptibility to drugs in culture,
- molecular genotyping.

6. ANTIMALARIAL TREATMENT POLICY

National antimalarial treatment policies should aim to offer antimalarials that are highly effective. The main determinant of policy change is the therapeutic efficacy and the consequent effectiveness of the antimalarial in use. Other important determinants include: changing patterns of malaria-associated morbidity and mortality; consumer and provider dissatisfaction with the current policy; and the availability of new products, strategies and approaches.

6.1   Assessment of *in vivo* therapeutic efficacy

This involves the assessment of clinical and parasitological outcomes of treatment over a certain period following the start of treatment, to check for the reappearance of parasites in the blood. Reappearance indicates reduced parasite sensitivity to the treatment drug. As a significant proportion of treatment failures do not appear until after day 14, shorter observation periods lead to a considerable overestimation of the efficacy of the tested drug. This is a particular problem at low levels of resistance and with low failure rates. The current recommended duration of follow-up is ≥28 days in areas of high as well as low to moderate transmission. Assessment over only 14 days, the period previously recommended in areas of high transmission, is no longer considered sufficient. Antimalarial treatment should also be assessed on the basis of parasitological cure rates. Where possible, blood or plasma levels of the antimalarial should also be measured in prospective assessments so that drug resistance can be distinguished from treatment failures due to pharmacokinetic reasons.

In high-transmission settings reinfection is inevitable, but cure of malaria (i.e. prevention of recrudescences) is important as it benefits both the patient, by reducing anaemia, and the community, by slowing the emergence and spread of resistance. In the past, "clinical" and "parasitological" cure rates were regarded separately, but with increasing appreciation of the adverse effects of treatment failure, the two are now considered together. Persistence of parasitaemia without fever following treatment has previously not been regarded seriously in high-transmission situations. This still represents a treatment failure and is associated with anaemia. Slowly eliminated antimalarials provide the additional benefit of suppressing malaria infections that are newly acquired during the period in which residual antimalarial drug levels persist in the body. On the other hand, these residual drug levels do provide a selection pressure for resistance. In these treatment recommendations, the curative efficacy of the antimalarials has taken precedence over these considerations.

6.2   Criteria for antimalarial treatment policy change

These malaria treatment guidelines recommend that antimalarial treatment policy should be changed at treatment failure rates considerably lower than those recommended previously. This major change reflects the availability of highly effective drugs, and the recognition both of the consequences of drug resistance, in terms of morbidity and mortality, and the importance of high cure rates in malaria control.

It is now recommended that a change of first-line treatment should be initiated if the total failure proportion exceeds 10%. However, it is acknowledged that a decision to change may be influenced by a number of additional factors, including the prevalence and geographical distribution of reported treatment failures, health service provider and/or patient dissatisfaction with the treatment, the political and economical context, and the availability of affordable alternatives to the commonly used treatment.

Summary of recommendations on changing antimalarial treatment policy

RECOMMENDATIONS	LEVEL OF EVIDENCE
In therapeutic efficacy assessments, the cure rate should be defined parasitologically, based on a minimum of 28 days of follow-up. Molecular genotyping using PCR technology should be used to distinguish recrudescent parasites from newly acquired infections.	E
Review and change of the antimalarial treatment policy should be initiated when the cure rate with the current recommended medicine falls below 90% (as assessed through monitoring of therapeutic efficacy).	E
A new recommended antimalarial medicine adopted as policy should have an average cure rate ≥ 95% as assessed in clinical trials.	E

7. TREATMENT OF UNCOMPLICATED
P. FALCIPARUM MALARIA[10]

7.1 Assessment

Uncomplicated malaria is defined as symptomatic malaria without signs of severity or evidence of vital organ dysfunction. In acute falciparum malaria there is a continuum from mild to severe malaria. Young children and non-immune adults with malaria may deteriorate rapidly. Detailed definitions of severe malaria are available (see section 8.1) to guide practitioners and for epidemiological and research purposes but, in practice, any patient whom the attending physician or health care worker suspects of having severe malaria should be treated as such initially. The risks of under-treating severe malaria considerably exceed those of giving parenteral or rectal treatment to a patient who does not need it.

7.2 Antimalarial combination therapy

To counter the threat of resistance of *P. falciparum* to monotherapies, and to improve treatment outcome, combinations of antimalarials are now recommended by WHO for the treatment of falciparum malaria.

7.2.1 Definition

Antimalarial combination therapy is the simultaneous use of two or more blood schizontocidal drugs with independent modes of action and thus unrelated biochemical targets in the parasite. The concept is based on the potential of two or more simultaneously administered schizontocidal drugs with independent modes of action to improve therapeutic efficacy and also to delay the development of resistance to the individual components of the combination.

7.2.2 What is not considered to be combination therapy

Drug combinations such as sulfadoxine–pyrimethamine, sulfalene–pyrimethamine, proguanil-dapsone, chlorproguanil-dapsone and atovaquone-proguanil rely on synergy between the two components. The drug targets in the malaria parasite are linked. These combinations are operationally considered as single products and treatment with them is not considered to be antimalarial combination therapy. Multiple-drug therapies that include a non-antimalarial medicine to enhance the antimalarial effect of a blood schizontocidal drug (e.g. chloroquine and chlorpheniramine) are also not antimalarial combination therapy.

---

[10] Further information is provided in Annex 7.

7.2.3   Rationale for antimalarial combination therapy

The rationale for combining antimalarials with different modes of action is twofold: (1) the combination is often more effective; and (2) in the rare event that a mutant parasite that is resistant to one of the drugs arises de novo during the course of the infection, the parasite will be killed by the other drug. This mutual protection is thought to prevent or delay the emergence of resistance. To realize the two advantages, the partner drugs in a combination must be independently effective. The possible disadvantages of combination treatments are the potential for increased risk of adverse effects and the increased cost.

7.2.4   Artemisinin-based combination therapy (ACT)

Artemisinin and its derivatives (artesunate, artemether, artemotil, dihydro-artemisinin) produce rapid clearance of parasitaemia and rapid resolution of symptoms. They reduce parasite numbers by a factor of approximately 10 000 in each asexual cycle, which is more than other current antimalarials (which reduce parasite numbers 100- to 1000-fold per cycle). Artemisinin and its derivatives are eliminated rapidly. When given in combination with rapidly eliminated compounds (tetracyclines, clindamycin), a 7-day course of treatment with an artemisinin compound is required; but when given in combination with slowly eliminated antimalarials, shorter courses of treatment (3 days) are effective. The evidence of their superiority in comparison to monotherapies has been clearly documented.

EVIDENCE: trials comparing monotherapies with ACTs[a]

Interventions: single drug (oral AQ, MQ or SP) compared with single drug in combination with AS (both oral)

Summary of RCTs: one meta-analysis of 11 RCTs has been conducted. This found a clear benefit of adding 3 days of AS to AQ, MQ or SP for uncomplicated malaria. The combination treatment resulted in fewer parasitological failures at day 28 and reduced gametocyte carriage compared to the baseline value. Adding AS treatment for 1 day (6 RCTs) was also associated with fewer treatment failures by day 28 but was significantly less effective than the 3-day regimen (OR: 0.34; 95% CI: 0.24–0.47; $p < 0.0001$).

Expert comment: the addition of AS to standard monotherapy significantly reduces treatment failure, recrudescence and gametocyte carriage.

Basis of decision: systematic review.

Recommendation: replace monotherapy with oral ACTs given for 3 days.

---

[a] See also Annex 7.1.

In 3-day ACT regimens, the artemisinin component is present in the body during only two asexual parasite life-cycles (each lasting 2 days, except for *P. malariae* infections). This exposure to 3 days of artemisinin treatment reduces the number of parasites in the body by a factor of approximately one hundred million ($10^4 \times 10^4 = 10^8$). However, complete clearance of parasites is dependent on the partner medicine being effective and persisting at parasiticidal concentrations until all the infecting parasites have been killed. Thus the partner compounds need to be relatively slowly eliminated. As a result of this the artemisinin component is "protected" from resistance by the partner medicine provided it is efficacious and the partner medicine is partly protected by the artemisinin derivative. Courses of ACTs of 1–2 days are not recommended; they are less efficacious, and provide less protection of the slowly eliminated partner antimalarial.

The artemisinin compounds are active against all four species of malaria parasites that infect humans and are generally well tolerated. The only significant adverse effect to emerge from extensive clinical trials has been rare (circa 1:3000) type 1 hypersensitivity reactions (manifested initially by urticaria). These drugs also have the advantage from a public health perspective of reducing gametocyte carriage and thus the transmissibility of malaria. This contributes to malaria control in areas of low endemicity.

7.2.5   Non-artemisinin based combination therapy

Non-artemisinin based combinations (non-ACTs) include sulfadoxine–pyrimethamine with chloroquine (SP+CQ) or amodiaquine (SP+AQ). However, the prevailing high levels of resistance have compromised the efficacy of these combinations. There is no convincing evidence that SP+CQ provides any additional benefit over SP, so this combination is not recommended; SP+AQ can be more effective than either drug alone, but needs to be considered in the light of comparison with ACTs. The evidence is summarized next page.

EVIDENCE: trials comparing monotherapies with non-ACTs[a]

Interventions: **oral SP+CQ compared with oral SP**

> *Summary of RCTs:* no RCTs with reported results for day 28 outcomes. Five subsequent RCTs found insufficient evidence of any difference in rates of treatment failure at days 14 and 21, respectively, between CQ+SP and SP alone, and gave no information on adverse events.
>
> *Expert comment:* increasing resistance to CQ in all settings means that neither of the options is recommended.
>
> *Basis of decision:* RCT.

Recommendation: do not use CQ+SP.

Interventions: **oral SP+AQ compared with oral AQ or oral SP**

> *Summary of RCTs:* one systematic review of SP+AQ compared with AQ alone with day 28 follow-up found no significant difference in day 28 outcomes.
>
> Three subsequent RCTs also found no significant differences in cure rates and levels of adverse events.
>
> One systematic review of SP+AQ compared with SP alone, found no significant difference in rates of day 28 cure or adverse events. One subsequent RCT found higher rates of day 28 cure and mid-adverse events with the combination compared to SP alone.
>
> *Expert comment:* in some areas where AQ+SP has been deployed, failure rates of this combination have increased rapidly.
>
> *Basis of decision:* systematic review.

Recommendation: if more effective medicines (ACTs) are not available and AQ and SP are effective,[b] AQ+SP may be used as an interim measure.

[a] See also Annex 7.2.

[b] Efficacy >80%.

> ## EVIDENCE: trials comparing ACTs with non-ACTs[a]
>
> *Interventions: oral ACTs compared with oral non-artesunate combinations*
>
> > *Summary of RCTs:* 1 RCT compared AS(for 3 days)+SP with AQ+SP. The total failure excluding new infections at day 28 was similar in the 2 groups (13% in the AS+SP group compared to 22% in the AQ+SP group; OR: 0.59; 95% CI: 0.29–1.18); total number of recurrent infections, including reinfections, was higher with AS+SP (29% with AS+SP, 17% with AQ+SP, OR: 0.49; 95% CI: 0.27–0.87).
> >
> > *Expert comment:* the above result is probably due to the efficacy of AQ that remains high, while SP failure is on the increase. In areas where AQ+SP has been adopted as first-line treatment, the impression is that there has been rapid development of resistance to AQ. This also makes both AQ and SP unavailable for use as an ACT component.
> >
> > *Basis of decision:* expert opinion.
>
> **Recommendation:** if more effective ACTs are not available and both AQ and SP are effective,[b] then AQ+SP may be used as an interim measure.

[a] See also Annex 7.3.

[b] Efficacy >80%.

7.3 The choice of artemisinin-based combination therapy options

Although there are some minor differences in oral absorption and bioavailability between the different artemisinin derivatives, there is no evidence that these differences are clinically significant in current formulations. It is the properties of the partner medicine that determine the effectiveness and choice of combination. ACTs with amodiaquine, atovaquone-proguanil, chloroquine, clindamycin, doxycycline, lumefantrine, mefloquine, piperaquine, pyronaridine, proguanil-dapsone, sulfadoxine–pyrimethamine and tetracycline have all been evaluated in trials carried out across the malaria-affected regions of the world. Some of these are studies for product development.

Though there are still gaps in our knowledge, there is reasonable evidence on safety and efficacy on which to base recommendations.

EVIDENCE: trials comparing ACTs[a]

Interventions: oral AL, AS+AQ, AS+MQ, AS+SP

> *Summary of RCTs:* AL 6-dose regimen compared with 4-dose regimen; 6 doses resulted in higher cure rate in 1 trial in Thailand (RR: 0.19; 95% CI: 0.06–0.62).
>
> AS+MQ compared with AL 6-dose regimen; systematic review including 2 small RCTs from Thailand. Higher proportion of patients with parasitaemia at day 28 with AL but difference not statistically significant. One additional RCT in Lao People's Democratic Republic also reported higher proportions of patients with parasitaemia at day 42 with AL but also not statistically significant.
>
> AS+AQ compared with AL 6-dose regimen; 1 trial in Tanzania found a significantly higher proportion of parasitological failures on day 28 with AS+AQ.
>
> No trials of AL compared with AS+SP.
>
> *Expert comment:* the efficacy of ACTs with AQ or SP as partner medicines is insufficient where cure rates with these medicines as monotherapies is less than 80%. The efficacy of AL and AS+MQ generally exceeds 90% except at the Thai-Cambodian border, where AL failure rate was 15%.
>
> *Basis of decision:* expert opinion.

Recommendations
1. Use the following ACTs: AL (6-dose regimen), AS+AQ, AS+MQ, AS+SP.
2. In areas with AQ and SP resistance exceeding 20% (PCR-corrected at day 28 of follow-up), use AS+MQ or AL.

[a] See also Annex 7.4

The following ACTs are currently recommended (alphabetical order):

- artemether-lumefantrine,
- artesunate + amodiaquine,
- artesunate + mefloquine,
- artesunate + sulfadoxine–pyrimethamine.

Note: amodiaquine + sulfadoxine–pyrimethamine may be considered as an interim option where ACTs cannot be made available, provided that efficacy of both is high.

7.3.1 Rationale for the exclusion of certain antimalarials

Several available drugs that were considered by the Technical Guidelines Development Group are currently not recommended.

- Chlorproguanil-dapsone has not yet been evaluated as an ACT partner drug, so there is insufficient evidence of both efficacy and safety to recommend it as a combination partner.

- Atovaquone-proguanil has been shown to be safe and effective as a combination partner in one large study, but is not included in these recommendations for deployment in endemic areas because of its very high cost.

- Halofantrine has not yet been evaluated as an ACT partner medicine and is not included in these recommendations because of safety concerns.

- Dihydroartemisinin (artenimol)-piperaquine has been shown to be safe and effective in large trials in Asia, but is not included in these recommendations as it is not yet available as a formulation manufactured under good manufacturing practices, and has not yet been evaluated sufficiently in Africa and South America.

Several other new antimalarial compounds are in development but do not yet have a sufficient clinical evidence to support recommendation here.

7.3.2 Deployment considerations affecting choice

Although for many countries, artemether-lumefantrine and artesunate + mefloquine may give the highest cure rates, there may be problems of affordability and availability of these products. Also, there is currently insufficient safety and tolerability data on artesunate + mefloquine at the recommended dose of 25mg/kg in African children to support its recommendation there. Trials with mefloquine monotherapy (25mg/kg) have raised concerns of tolerability in African children. Countries may therefore opt instead to use artesunate + amodiaquine and artesunate + sulfadoxine–pyrimethamine, which may have lower cure rates because of resistance. Although still effective in some areas, sulfadoxine–pyrimethamine and amodiaquine are widely available as monotherapies, providing continued selection pressure, and it is likely that resistance will continue to worsen despite deployment of the corresponding ACTs. This may be a particular problem in settings where sulfadoxine–pyrimethamine is being used for intermittent preventive treatment in pregnancy; artesunate + sulfadoxine–pyrimethamine should probably not be used in such settings.

Summary of recommendations on treatment for uncomplicated falciparum malaria

RECOMMENDATIONS	LEVEL OF EVIDENCE
The treatment of choice for uncomplicated falciparum malaria is a combination of two or more antimalarials with different mechanisms of action.	S, T, O
ACTs are the recommended treatments for uncomplicated falciparum malaria.	S
The following ACTs are currently recommended:	S, T, O
– artemether-lumefantrine, artesunate + amodiaquine, artesunate + mefloquine, artesunate + sulfadoxine-pyrimethamine.	
The choice of ACT in a country or region will be based on the level of resistance of the partner medicine in the combination:	
– in areas of multidrug resistance (South-East Asia), artesunate + mefloquine or artemether-lumefantrine	E
– in Africa, artemether-lumefantrine, artesunate + amodiaquine; artesunate + sulfadoxine-pyrimethamine.	S
The artemisinin derivative components of the combination must be given for at least 3 days for an optimum effect.	S
Artemether-lumefantrine should be used with a 6-dose regimen.	T, E
Amodiaquine + sulfadoxine-pyrimethamine may be considered as an interim option in situations where ACTs cannot be made available.	E

7.4   Practical aspects of treatment with recommended ACTs

7.4.1   Artemether-lumefantrine

This is currently available as co-formulated tablets containing 20 mg of artemether and 120 mg of lumefantrine. The total recommended treatment is a 6-dose regimen of artemether-lumefantrine twice a day for 3 days.

Table 1.   **Dosing schedule for artemether-lumefantrine**

Body weight in kg	No. of tablets at approximate timing of dosing[a]					
(age in years)	0 h	8 h	24 h	36 h	48 h	60 h
5–14 (<3)	1	1	1	1	1	1
15–24 (≥3–8)	2	2	2	2	2	2
25–34 (≥9–14)	3	3	3	3	3	3
>34 (>14)	4	4	4	4	4	4

[a] The regimen can be expressed more simply for ease of use at the programme level as follows: the second dose on the first day should be given any time between 8 h and 12 h after the first dose. Dosage on the second and third days is twice a day (morning and evening).

An advantage of this combination is that lumefantrine is not available as a monotherapy and has never been used by itself for the treatment of malaria. Recent evidence indicates that the therapeutic response and safety profile in young children of less than 10 kg is similar to that in older children, and artemether-lumefantrine is now recommended for patients ≥ 5 kg. Lumefantrine absorption is enhanced by co-administration with fat. Low blood levels, with resultant treatment failure, could potentially result from inadequate fat intake, and so it is essential that patients or carers are informed of the need to take this ACT with milk or fat-containing food – particularly on the second and third days of treatment.

7.4.2   Artesunate + amodiaquine

This is currently available as separate scored tablets containing 50 mg of artesunate and 153 mg base of amodiaquine, respectively. Co-formulated tablets are under development. The total recommended treatment is 4 mg/kg bw of artesunate and 10 mg base/kg bw of amodiaquine given once a day for 3 days.

Table 2.   **Dosing schedule for artesunate + amodiaquine**

	Dose in mg (No. of tablets)					
Age	Artesunate (50 mg)			Amodiaquine (153 mg)		
	Day 1	Day 2	Day 3	Day 1	Day 2	Day 3
5–11 months	25 (½)	25	25	76 (½)	76	76
≥1–6 years	50 (1)	50	50	153 (1)	153	153
≥7–13 years	100 (2)	100	100	306 (2)	306	306
>13 years	200 (4)	200	200	612 (4)	612	612

This combination is sufficiently efficacious only where 28-day cure rates with amodiaquine monotherapy exceed 80%. Resistance is likely to worsen with continued availability of chloroquine and amodiaquine monotherapies. More information on the safety of artesunate + amodiaquine is needed from prospective pharmacovigilance programmes.

7.4.3   Artesunate + sulfadoxine–pyrimethamine

This is currently available as separate scored tablets containing 50 mg of artesunate, and tablets containing 500 mg of sulfadoxine and 25 mg of pyri-methamine.[11] The total recommended treatment is 4 mg/kg bw of artesunate given once a day for 3 days and a single administration of sulfadoxine-pyrimethamine (25/1.25 mg base/kg bw) on day 1.

Table 3.   **Dosing schedule for artesunate + sulfadoxine-pyrimethamine**

Age	Dose in mg (No. of tablets)					
	Artesunate (50 mg)			Sulfadoxine-pyrimethamine (500/25)		
	Day 1	Day 2	Day 3	Day 1	Day 2	Day 3
5–11 months	25 (¹/₂)	25	25	250/12.5 (¹/₂)	–	–
≥1–6 years	50 (1)	50	50	500/25 (1)	–	–
≥7–13 years	100 (2)	100	100	1000/50 (2)	–	–
>13 years	200 (4)	200	200	1500/75 (3)	–	–

While a single dose of sulfadoxine–pyrimethamine is sufficient, it is necessary for artesunate to be given for 3 days for satisfactory efficacy. This combination is sufficiently efficacious only where 28-day cure rates with sulfadoxine–pyrimethamine alone exceed 80%. Resistance is likely to worsen with continued availability of sulfadoxine–pyrimethamine, sulfalene–pyrimethamine and cotrimoxazole (trimethoprim-sulfamethoxazole).

7.4.4   Artesunate + mefloquine

This is currently available as separate scored tablets containing 50 mg of artesunate and 250 mg base of mefloquine, respectively. Co-formulated tablets are under development but are not available at present. The total recommended treatment is 4 mg/kg bw of artesunate given once a day for 3 days and 25 mg base/kg bw of mefloquine usually split over 2 or 3 days.

---

[11] A similar medicine with tablets containing 500 mg of sulfalene and 25 mg of pyrimethamine is considered to be equivalent to sulfadoxine-pyrimethamine.

Table 4. **Dosing schedule for artesunate + mefloquine**

Age	Dose in mg (No. of tablets)					
	Artesunate (50 mg)			Mefloquine (250 mg)		
	Day 1	Day 2	Day 3	Day 1	Day 2	Day 3
5–11 months	25 (½)	25	25	–	125 (½)	–
≥1–6 years	50 (1)	50	50	–	250 (1)	–
≥7–13 years	100 (2)	100	100	–	500 (2)	250 (1)
>13 years	200 (4)	200	200	–	1000 (4)	500 (2)

Two different doses of mefloquine have been evaluated, 15 mg base/kg bw and 25 mg base/kg bw. The lower dose is associated with inferior efficacy and is not recommended. To reduce acute vomiting and optimize absorption, the 25 mg/kg dose is usually split and given either as 15 mg/kg (usually on the second day) followed by 10 mg/kg one day later, or as 8.3 mg/kg per day for 3 days. Pending development of a co-formulated product, malaria control programmes will have to decide on the optimum operational strategy of mefloquine dosing for their populations. Mefloquine is associated with an increased incidence of nausea, vomiting, dizziness, dysphoria and sleep disturbance in clinical trials, but these are seldom debilitating and in general, where this ACT has been deployed, it has been well tolerated.

7.5   Incorrect approaches to treatment

In endemic regions, some semi-immune malaria patients could be cured using partial treatment with effective medicines (i.e. use of regimens that would be unsatisfactory in patients with no immunity). This had led in the past to different recommendations for patients considered to be semi-immune and those considered to be non-immune. Another potentially dangerous practice is to give only the first dose of the treatment course for patients with suspected but unconfirmed malaria, with the intention of giving full treatment if the diagnosis is eventually confirmed. Neither practice is recommended. If malaria is suspected and the decision to treat is made, then a full effective treatment is required whether or not the diagnosis is confirmed by a test.

With the exception of artemether-lumefantrine, the partner medicines of all other ACTs have been previously used as monotherapies, and still continue to be available as such in many countries. Their continued use as monotherapies can potentially compromise the value of ACTs by selecting for drug resistance. The withdrawal of artemisinins and other monotherapies is recommended.

Summary of recommendations on treatment approaches that should be avoided

RECOMMENDATIONS	LEVEL OF EVIDENCE
Partial treatments should not be given even when patients are considered to be semi-immune or the diagnosis is uncertain. A full course of effective treatment should always be given once a decision to give antimalarial treatment has been reached.	E
The artemisinins and partner medicines of ACTs should not be available as monotherapies.	E

7.6   Additional aspects of clinical management

7.6.1   Can the patient take oral medication?

Some patients cannot tolerate oral treatment, and will require parenteral or rectal administration for 1–2 days until they can swallow and retain oral medication reliably. Although such patients may not show signs of severity, they should receive the same antimalarial dose regimens as for severe malaria (see section 8.4).

7.6.2   Does the patient have very high parasitaemia (hyperparasitaemia)?

Some patients may have no signs of severity but on examination of the blood film are found to have very high parasitaemia. The risks associated with high parasitaemia vary depending on the age of the patient and on transmission intensity. Thus cut-off values and definitions of hyperparasitaemia also vary. Patients with high parasitaemias are at an increased risk of treatment failure and of developing severe malaria, and therefore have an increased risk of dying. These patients can be treated with the oral ACTs recommended for uncomplicated malaria. However, they require close monitoring to ensure that the drugs are retained and that signs of severity do not develop, and they may require a longer course of treatment to ensure cure. Details of definitions and management are provided in sections 8.1 and 8.15.

7.6.3   Use of antipyretics

Fever is a cardinal feature of malaria, and is associated with constitutional symptoms of lassitude, weakness, headache, anorexia and often nausea. In young children, high fevers are associated with vomiting, including of medication, and seizures. Treatment is with antipyretics and, if necessary, tepid sponging. Care should be taken to ensure that the water is not too cool as, paradoxically, this may raise the core temperature by inducing cutaneous vasoconstriction. Paracetamol (acetaminophen) 15 mg/kg bw every 4 h is widely used; it is safe and well tolerated given orally or as a suppository. Ibuprofen (5 mg/kg bw) has been used successfully as an alternative in malaria and other childhood fevers, although there is less experience with this compound. Acetylsalicylic acid (aspirin) should not be used in children because of the risks of Reye's syndrome. There has been some concern that antipyretics might attenuate the host defence against malaria, as their use is associated with delayed parasite clearance. However, this appears to result from delaying cytoadherence, which is likely to be beneficial. There is no reason to withhold antipyretics in malaria.

EVIDENCE: trials of routine use of antipyretics in uncomplicated falciparum malaria

Interventions: oral paracetamol, oral nonsteroidal antiinflammatory drugs, mechanical methods

> *Summary of RCTs:* a systematic review of 12 trials (*n* = 1509) in children using paracetamol.
>
> Systematic review of 3 randomised trials in adults did not provide any evidence that antipyretic medicines prolonged illness.
>
> In 2 trials, where all children received an antipyretic medicine, physical methods resulted in a higher proportion of children without fever at one hour (*n* = 125, RR: 11.76; 95% CI: 3.39–40.79). In a third trial (*n* = 130), which only reported mean change in temperature, no difference was detected.
>
> *Expert comment:* symptomatic treatment of fever is indicated and is particularly important in small children in whom fever can cause seizures and induce vomiting (more likely if core temperature is >38 °C). Mechanical antipyretic measures, such as exposure and fanning cause a transient reduction in temperature, oral antipyretics may be more effective for reducing temperature.

Recommendation: use paracetamol or ibuprofen for treating fever (particularly if temperature is > 38.5 °C). Mechanical methods have an additive effect.

Summary of recommendations on management of fever

RECOMMENDATIONS	LEVEL OF EVIDENCE
An antipyretic medicine and physical methods for fever reduction should be administered to children with fever. This is particularly important in children when core temperature is ≥ 38.5 °C.	S, E
Paracetamol (acetaminophen) and ibuprofen are the preferred options for reducing fever.	S, E

7.6.4   Use of antiemetics

Vomiting is common in acute malaria and may be severe. Antiemetics are widely used. There have been no studies of their efficacy in malaria, and no comparisons between different antiemetic compounds, although there is no evidence that they are harmful.

7.6.5   Management of seizures

Generalized seizures are more common in children with falciparum malaria than in those with the other malarias. This suggests an overlap between the cerebral pathology resulting from malaria and febrile convulsions. Sometimes these seizures are the prodrome of cerebral malaria. If the seizure is ongoing, the airway should be maintained and anticonvulsants given (parenteral or rectal benzodiazepines or intramuscular paraldehyde). If it has stopped, the child should be treated as indicated in section 7.6.3 if core temperature is above 38.5 °C. There is no evidence that prophylactic anticonvulsants are beneficial in otherwise uncomplicated malaria.

7.7   Operational issues in treatment management

To optimize the benefit of deploying ACTs, and to have an impact on malaria, it will be necessary to deploy them as widely as possible – this means at most peripheral health clinics and health centres, and in the community. Deployment through the formal public health delivery system alone will not reach many of those who need treatment. In several countries, they must also be available through the private sector. Ultimately, effective treatment needs to be available at community or household level in such a way that there is no financial or physical barrier to access. The strategy to secure full access must be based on an analysis of the national and local health systems, and will often require adjustment based on programme monitoring and operational research. The dissemination of clear national treatment guidelines, use of appropriate information, education and communication materials, monitoring both of the deployment process, access and coverage and provision of adequately packaged and presented antimalarials are needed to optimize the benefits of providing these new effective treatments widely.

7.7.1   Health education

At all levels, from the hospital to the community, education is vital to optimizing antimalarial treatment. Clear guidelines in the language understood by the local users, posters, wall charts, educational videos and other teaching materials, public awareness campaigns, education of and provision of information materials to shopkeepers and other dispensers can all improve the understanding of malaria and the likelihood of improved prescribing and adherence, appropriate referral, and minimizing the unnecessary use of antimalarials.

7.7.2 Adherence to treatment

To achieve the desired therapeutic effectiveness, a drug must be intrinsically efficacious and must be taken in the correct doses at the proper intervals. Patient adherence is a major determinant of the response to antimalarials, as most treatments are taken at home without medical supervision. There have been few studies of adherence. These suggest that 3-day regimens of medicines such as ACTs are adhered to reasonably well, provided that patients or carers are given an adequate explanation at the time of prescribing. Prescribers, shopkeepers or vendors should therefore give a clear and comprehensible explanation of how to use the medicines. Co-formulation is probably a very important contributor to adherence. User-friendly packaging, such as blister packs, also encourage completion of the treatment course and correct dosing.

7.7.3 Quality assurance of antimalarial medicines

Many of the antimalarials available in malaria endemic areas are substandard in that the manufacturing processes have been unsatisfactory, or their pharmaceutical properties do not meet the required pharmacopoeial specifications. Counterfeit tablets and ampoules containing no antimalarials are a major problem in some areas. These may result in fatal delays in appropriate treatment, and may also give rise to a mistaken impression of resistance. WHO, in collaboration with other United Nations agencies, has established an international mechanism to pre-qualify manufacturers of artemisinin compounds and ACTs on the basis of compliance with internationally-recommended standards of manufacturing and quality. It is the responsibility of national ministries of Health and regulatory authorities to ensure the quality of antimalarials provided through both the public and private sectors, through regulation, inspection and law enforcement.

7.7.4 Pharmacovigilance

Rare but serious adverse effects are often not detected in clinical trials and can only be detected through pharmacovigilance systems operating in situations of wide population use. There are few data from prospective Phase IV post-marketing studies on rare but potentially serious adverse effects of antimalarials. Chloroquine has the best-documented adverse effect profile. The safety profiles of the artemisinin derivatives, mefloquine and sulfadoxine–pyrimethamine are supported by a reasonable evidence base, but mainly from large clinical trials.

The neurotoxicity observed in animals treated with artemisinin derivatives has prompted large prospective assessments in humans, but no evidence of neurotoxicity has been found. Concerns over the risk of severe liver or skin reactions to sulfadoxine-pyrimethamine treatment have receded with increasing numbers of negative reports. More data are needed on the newer drugs and on amodiaquine as well. There is also an urgent need to obtain more information on the safety of antimalarials, in particular the ACTs, in pregnancy. It is recommended that countries or regions should consider establishing pharmacovigilance systems if they have not already done so.

7.8   Management of treatment failures

7.8.1   Failure within 14 days

Treatment failure within 14 days of receiving an ACT is very unusual. Of 39 trials of artemisinin or its derivatives, which together enrolled 6124 patients, 32 trials (4917 patients) had no failures at all by day 14. In the remaining 7 trials, failure rates at day 14 ranged from 1% to 7%. The majority of treatment failures occur after 2 weeks of initial treatment. In many cases failures are missed because patients presenting with malaria are not asked whether they have received antimalarial treatment within the preceding 1–2 months. Recurrence of falciparum malaria can be the result of a reinfection, or a recrudescence (i.e. failure). In an individual patient it may not be possible to distinguish recrudescence from reinfection, although if fever and parasitaemia fail to resolve or recur within 2 weeks of treatment then this is considered a failure of treatment. Wherever possible treatment failure must be confirmed parasitologically – preferably by blood slide examination (as HRP2-based tests may remain positive for weeks after the initial infection even without recrudescence). This may require transferring the patient to a facility with microscopy; transfer may be necessary anyway to obtain second-line treatment. Treatment failures may result from drug resistance, poor adherence or unusual pharmacokinetic properties in that individual. It is important to determine from the patient's history whether he or she vomited previous treatment or did not complete a full course. Treatment failures within 14 days should be treated with a second-line antimalarial (see section 7.8.3).

7.8.2   Failure after 14 days

Recurrence of fever and parasitaemia more than 2 weeks after treatment, which could result either from recrudescence or new infection, can be retreated with the first-line ACT. Parasitological confirmation is desirable but not a precondition. If it is a recrudescence, then the first-line treatment should still be effective in most cases. This simplifies operational management and drug deployment. However, reuse of mefloquine within 28 days of first treatment is associated with an increased risk of neuropsychiatric sequelae and, in this particular case, second-line treatment should be given. If there is a further recurrence, then malaria should be confirmed parasitologically and second-line treatment given.

7.8.3 Recommended second-line antimalarial treatments

On the basis of the evidence from current practice and the consensus opinion of the Guidelines Development Group, the following second-line treatments are recommended, in order of preference:

- alternative ACT known to be effective in the region,
- artesunate + tetracycline or doxycycline or clindamycin,
- quinine + tetracycline or doxycycline or clindamycin.

The alternative ACT has the advantages of simplicity, and where available, co-formulation to improve adherence. The 7-day quinine regimes are not well tolerated and adherence is likely to be poor if treatment is not observed.

Summary of recommendations on second-line antimalarial treatment for uncomplicated falciparum malaria

RECOMMENDATIONS	LEVEL OF EVIDENCE
Alternative ACT known to be effective in the region.	O
Artesunate (2 mg/kg bw once a day) + tetracycline (4 mg/kg bw four times a day) or doxycycline (3.5 mg/kg bw once a day) or clindamycin (10 mg/kg bw twice a day). Any of these combinations to be given for 7 days.	O
Quinine (10 mg salt/kg bw three times a day) + tetracycline or doxycycline or clindamycin. Any of these combinations to be given for 7 days.	O

7.9   Treatment in specific populations and situations

7.9.1 Pregnant women

Pregnant women with symptomatic acute malaria are a high-risk group, and must receive effective antimalarials. Malaria in pregnancy is associated with low birth weight, increased anaemia and, in low-transmission areas, an increased risk of severe malaria. In high-transmission settings, despite the adverse effects on fetal growth, malaria is usually asymptomatic in pregnancy. There is insufficient information on the safety and efficacy of most antimalarials in pregnancy, particularly for exposure in the first trimester, and so treatment recommendations are different to those for non-pregnant adults. Organogenesis occurs mainly in the first trimester and this is therefore the time of greatest concern for potential teratogenicity, although nervous system development continues throughout pregnancy. The antimalarials considered safe in the first trimester of pregnancy are quinine, chloroquine, proguanil, pyrimethamine and sulfadoxine–pyrimethamine. Of these, quinine remains the most effective and can be used in all trimesters of pregnancy including the first trimester. In reality women often do not declare their pregnancies in the first trimester and so, early pregnancies will often be exposed inadvertently to the available first-line treatment. Inadvertent exposure to antimalarials is not an indication for termination of the pregnancy.

There is increasing experience with artemisinin derivatives in the second and third trimesters (over 1000 documented pregnancies). There have been no adverse effects on the mother or fetus. The current assessment of benefits compared with potential risks suggests that the artemisinin derivatives should be used to treat uncomplicated falciparum malaria in the second and third trimesters of pregnancy, but should not be used in the first trimester until more information becomes available. The choice of combination partner is difficult. Mefloquine has been associated with an increased risk of stillbirth in large observational studies in Thailand, but not in Malawi. Amodiaquine, chlorpro-guanil-dapsone, halofantrine, lumefantrine and piperaquine have not been evaluated sufficiently to permit positive recommendations. Sulfadoxine–pyrimethamine is safe but may be ineffective in many areas because of increasing resistance. Clindamycin is also safe, but both medicines (clindamycin and the artemisinin partner) must be given for 7 days. Primaquine and tetra-cyclines should not be used in pregnancy.

Despite these many uncertainties, effective treatment must not be delayed in pregnant women. Given the disadvantages of quinine, i.e. the long course of treatment, and the increased risk of hypoglycaemia in the second and third trimesters, ACTs are considered suitable alternatives for these trimesters. In practice, if first-line treatment with an artemisinin combination is all that is immediately available to treat in the first trimester of pregnancy pregnant women who have symptomatic malaria, then this should be given. Pharmaco-vigilance programmes to document the outcome of pregnancies where there has been exposure to ACTs, and if possible documentation of the development of the infant, are encouraged so that future recommendations can stand on a firmer footing.

EVIDENCE: trials on the use of antimalarial medicines for the treatment of uncomplicated malaria in pregnant women

Interventions: oral AS+MQ, oral CQ alone, oral quinine, oral quinine + clindamycin

> *Summary of RCTs:* four randomized and two quasi-randomized trials with 513 pregnant participants. There were fewer treatment failures with AS+MQ than with quinine in one trial (day 63: RR: 0.09; 95% CI: 0.02–0.38; 106 participants). Data for other comparisons are scant. Where trials reported adverse outcomes, there were no differences reported between treatments in terms of effect on the mother or the fetus.
>
> *Expert comment:* systematic summaries of safety suggest that the artemisinin derivatives are safe in the second and third trimesters of pregnancy. One large observational study in Thailand suggests an increased risk of stillbirth associated with MQ but this was not found in a study conducted in Malawi. There are as yet insufficient safety data about the use of artemisinin derivatives in the first trimester of pregnancy.
>
> *Basis of decision:* expert opinion.

Recommendations: for the first trimester of pregnancy: quinine +/– clindamycin.

For second and third trimesters:
1. the ACT being used in the country/region, or
2. artesunate + clindamycin,
3. quinine + clindamycin.

Summary of recommendations on the treatment of uncomplicated falciparum malaria in pregnancy

RECOMMENDATIONS	LEVEL OF EVIDENCE
First trimester: quinine + clindamycin[a] to be given for 7 days. ACT should be used if it is the only effective treatment available.	O, E
Second and third trimesters: ACT known to be effective in the country/region or artesunate + clindamycin to be given for 7 days or quinine + clindamycin to be given for 7 days.	O, E

[a] If clindamycin is unavailable or unaffordable, then the monotherapy should be given.

7.9.2   Lactating women

The amounts of antimalarials that enter breast milk and are therefore likely to be consumed by the breast-feeding infant are relatively small. The only exception to this is dapsone, relatively large amounts of which are excreted in breast milk (14% of the adult dose), and pending further data this should not be prescribed. Tetracyclines are also contraindicated because of their effect on the infant's bones and teeth.

Summary of recommendations on the treatment of uncomplicated falciparum malaria in lactating women

RECOMMENDATION	LEVEL OF EVIDENCE
Lactating women should receive standard antimalarial treatment (including ACTs) except for tetracyclines and dapsone, which should be withheld during lactation.	E

7.9.3   Infants[12]

Choice of antimalarial drug

In endemic countries, malaria is common in infants and children under 2 years of age. Immunity acquired from the mother wanes after 3–6 months of age, and the case-fatality rate of severe malaria in infants is higher than in older children. Furthermore, there are important differences between infants and older children in the pharmacokinetics of many medicines. Accurate dosing is particularly important in infants. Despite this, few clinical studies focus specifically on this age range, partly because of ethical considerations relating to the recruitment of very young children to clinical trials, and also because of the difficulty of repeated blood sampling. In the majority of clinical studies, subgroup analysis is not used to distinguish between infants and older children. Infants are more likely to vomit or regurgitate antimalarial treatment than older children or adults. Taste, volume, consistency and gastrointestinal tolerability are important determinants of whether the child retains the treatment. Mothers often need advice on techniques of medicine administration and the importance of administering the medicine again if it is immediately regurgitated. With the increasing failure of chloroquine and sulfadoxine–pyrimethamine as front-line antimalarials, the challenge is now to find safe alternatives in this age group. Fortunately the artemisinin derivatives appear to be safe in, and well tolerated by young children, and so the choice of ACT will be determined largely by the safety and tolerability of the partner drug. The limited information available does not indicate particular problems with currently recommended ACTs in infancy.

Dosing

Although dosing based on body area is recommended for many drugs in young children, for the sake of simplicity, dosing of antimalarials has been traditionally based on weight. The weight-adjusted doses of antimalarials in

---

[12] A detailed review of the available data on safety of antimalarials in infants is provided in Annex 3, section A3.17.

infants are similar to those used in adults. For the majority of antimalarials, however, the lack of an infant formulation necessitates the division of adult tablets, which leads to inaccurate dosing. There is a need to develop infant formulations for a range of antimalarials in order to improve the accuracy and reliability of dosing.

Delay in treating falciparum malaria may have fatal consequences, particularly for more severe infections. Every effort should be made to give oral treatment and ensure that it is retained. In situations where it is not possible to give parenteral treatment, a sick infant who vomits antimalarial medicine treatment repeatedly, has a seizure or is too weak to swallow reliably should be given artesunate by the rectal route, pending transfer to a facility where parenteral treatment is possible. Large trials assessing the impact of this strategy on mortality have recently been undertaken in remote rural areas, but results are not yet available. Pharmacological and trial evidence concerning the rectal administration of artesunate and other antimalarial drugs is provided in section 8.7.

Summary of recommendations on treatment of uncomplicated falciparum malaria in infants and young children

RECOMMENDATIONS	LEVEL OF EVIDENCE
The acutely ill child requires careful clinical monitoring as they may deteriorate rapidly.	E
ACTs should be used as first-line treatment for infants and young children.	T, O, E
Referral to a health centre or hospital is indicated for young children who cannot swallow antimalarials reliably.	E

7.9.4 Travellers

Travellers who acquire malaria are often non-immune adults either from cities with little or no transmission within endemic countries, or visitors from non-endemic countries. Both are likely to be at a higher risk of malaria and its consequences because they have no immunity to malaria. Within the malaria endemic country they should in principle be treated according to national policy. Travellers who return to a non-endemic country and then develop malaria present particular problems and, have a high case fatality rate. Doctors may be unfamiliar with malaria and the diagnosis may be delayed, relevant antimalarials may not be registered and/or therefore available. If the patient falls ill far from a major health facility, availability of antimalarials can be a life-threatening issue despite registration. On the other hand prevention of emergence of resistance and transmission are of less relevance outside malaria endemic areas. Thus monotherapy may be given if it can be assured to be effective. Furthermore cost of treatment is usually not a limiting factor. The principles underlying the recommendations given below are that effective medicines should be used to treat travellers; if the patient has taken chemoprophylaxis, then the same medicine should not be used for treatment. The treatment for *P. vivax*, *P. ovale* and *P. malariae* in travellers should be the same as for these infections in patients from endemic areas (see section 9).

In the management of severe malaria outside endemic areas, there may be delays in obtaining artesunate, artemether or quinine. If parenteral quinidine is available but other parenteral drugs are not, then this should be given with careful clinical and electrocardiographic monitoring (see section 8).

EVIDENCE: treatment of uncomplicated malaria in travellers returning to non-endemic areas

Interventions: atovaquone–proguanil, halofantrine, quinine, quinine + clindamycin, artemether-lumefantrine

> *Summary of RCTs:* three RCTS (total 259 patients) report effective treatment with all interventions listed although the artemether-lumefantrine regimen was only 4 doses and therefore less effective. In one trial using halofantrine significant prolongation of the QT interval was noted.
>
> *Expert comment:* halofantrine is not recommended because of significant cardiotoxicity compared to other treatments.
>
> *Basis of decision:* RCTs and expert opinion.

Recommendation: the following antimalarials are suitable for use in travellers returning to non-endemic countries:
- artemether-lumefantrine (6-dose regimen),
- atovaquone–proguanil,
- quinine + doxycycline or clindamycin.

Summary of recommendations on the treatment of falciparum malaria in non-immune travellers

RECOMMENDATIONS	LEVEL OF EVIDENCE
For travellers returning to non-endemic countries:[a]	O, E
– atovaquone–proguanil (15/6 mg/kg, usual adult dose, 4 tablets once a day for 3 days);	
– artemether–lumefantrine (adult dose, 4 tablets twice a day for 3 days);	
– quinine (10 mg salt/kg bw every 8 h) + doxycycline[b] (3.5 mg/kg bw once a day) or clindamycin (10 mg/kg bw twice a day); all drugs to be given for 7 days	
For severe malaria:	O, E
– the antimalarial treatment of severe malaria in travellers is the same as shown in section 8;	
– travellers with severe malaria should be managed in an intensive care unit;	
– haemofiltration or haemodialysis should be started early in acute renal failure or severe metabolic acidosis;	
– positive pressure ventilation should be started early if there is any breathing pattern abnormality, intractable seizure or acute respiratory distress syndrome.	

[a] Halofantrine is not recommended as first-line treatment for uncomplicated malaria because of cardiotoxicity.

[b] Doxycycline should not be used in children under 8 years of age.

7.10 Coexisting morbidities

7.10.1 HIV infection[13]

Increasing numbers of people in malaria endemic areas are living with HIV infection. It is becoming increasingly apparent that, as HIV progresses and immunosuppression worsens, the manifestations of malaria also worsen. In pregnant women, the adverse effects on birth weight are increased. In patients with partial immunity to malaria, the severity of the infection is increased. There is insufficient information at the present time on how HIV infection modifies the therapeutic response to antimalarials. However, increasing parasite burdens and reduced host immunity, both of which occur with HIV infection, are associated with increased treatment failure rates. At this time, there is insufficient

---

[13] Further information on malaria treatment and HIV/AIDS is provided in Annex 8.

information to modify the general malaria treatment recommendations for patients with HIV/AIDS. Current UNAIDS/WHO recommendations on the prophylaxis of opportunistic infections with cotrimoxazole (trimethoprim-sulfamethoxazole) in people living with HIV/AIDS remain unchanged (see below). However, treatment with sulfadoxine–pyrimethamine should not be given to patients on cotrimoxazole as there is probably an increased risk of sulfa-related adverse effects (and in any case as both medicines have similar antimalarial activity, the malaria infection is likely to be resistant to sulfadoxine–pyrimethamine). Depending on the malaria transmission setting, HIV-infected individuals are at increased risk of asymptomatic parasitaemia, clinical malaria or severe and complicated malaria. Therefore, they have an even greater need for malaria control measures than individuals not infected with HIV.

EVIDENCE: treatment of malaria in patients co-infected with HIV

Interventions: **oral ACTs, oral SP**

Summary of RCTs: none.

Expert comment: observational studies suggest that malaria is more severe in patients co-infected with HIV. There is concern that severe adverse reactions to sulfonamides may be more frequent in HIV patients receiving cotrimoxazole (trimethoprim-sulfamethoxazole) for prophylaxis against opportunistic infections who are treated with SP for malaria.

Basis of decision: expert opinion.

Recommendation: there is insufficient evidence to recommend modifications to antimalarial treatment regimens in patients infected with HIV.

SP should be avoided for malaria treatment in HIV-infected patients receiving cotrimoxazole prophylaxis.

Summary of the recommendations on treatment of uncomplicated falciparum malaria in patients with HIV infection

RECOMMENDATIONS	LEVEL OF EVIDENCE
Patients with HIV infection who develop malaria should receive standard antimalarial treatment regimens as recommended in the relevant sections of the guidelines.	E
Treatment or intermittent preventive treatment with sulfadoxine-pyrimethamine should not be given to HIV-infected patients receiving cotrimoxazole (trimethoprim-sulfamethoxazole) prophylaxis.	E

7.10.2 Severe malnutrition

Malaria and malnutrition frequently coexist. There are only a few studies of antimalarial medicine disposition in people with malnutrition, although many antimalarial drug efficacy studies have been conducted in populations and settings where malnutrition was prevalent (see Annex 3, section A3.17.2).

Changes in drug kinetics in malnutrition

Drug absorption may be reduced owing to diarrhoea and vomiting, rapid gut transit and atrophy of the bowel mucosa. Absorption of intramuscular and possibly intrarectal drugs may be slower and diminished muscle mass may make it difficult to administer repeated intramuscular injections. The volume of distribution of some drugs would be expected to be larger and plasma concentrations lower. Hypoalbuminaemia, resulting from decreased synthesis as dietary deficiency occurs, could lead to an increase in the concentration of unbound drug; this may increase metabolic clearance, but hepatic dysfunction may reduce the metabolism of some drugs.

Antimalarial drugs and protein energy malnutrition

There are limited studies of the effect of malnutrition on chloroquine, doxycycline, quinine, sulfadoxine–pyrimethamine and tetracycline, and not all of these studies were conducted in patients with malaria. There is insufficient evidence to suggest that the dosages in mg/kg bw of any antimalarial should be changed in patients with malnutrition.

There are no studies in malnourished patients of amodiaquine, artemisinin derivatives, artemether-lumefantrine, atovaquone–proguanil, clindamycin, mefloquine or primaquine.

Summary of the recommendations on treatment of uncomplicated falciparum malaria in malnourished patients

RECOMMENDATION	LEVEL OF EVIDENCE
Although there are many reasons why drug kinetics may be different in malnourished patients as compared with those who are well nourished, there is insufficient evidence to change current mg/kg bw dosing recommendations.	E

8. TREATMENT OF SEVERE FALCIPARUM MALARIA[14]

8.1 Definition

In a patient with *P. falciparum* asexual parasitaemia and no other obvious cause of their symptoms, the presence of one or more of the following clinical or laboratory features classifies the patient as suffering from severe malaria[15]:

Clinical manifestation:
- Prostration
- Impaired consciousness
- Respiratory distress (acidotic breathing)
- Multiple convulsions
- Circulatory collapse
- Pulmonary oedema (radiological)
- Abnormal bleeding
- Jaundice
- Haemoglobinuria

Laboratory test:
- Severe anaemia
- Hypoglycaemia
- Acidosis
- Renal impairment
- Hyperlactataemia
- Hyperparasitaemia

8.2 Treatment objectives

The main objective is to prevent the patient from dying, secondary objectives are prevention of recrudescence, transmission or emergence of resistance and prevention of disabilities.

The mortality of untreated severe malaria is thought to approach 100%. With anti-malarial treatment the mortality falls to 15–20% overall, although within the broad definition are syndromes associated with mortality rates that are lower (e.g. severe anaemia) and higher (metabolic acidosis). Death from severe malaria often occurs within hours of admission to hospital or clinic, and so it is essential that therapeutic concentrations of antimalarial are achieved as soon as possible.

---

[14] Further information is provided in Annex 9.

[15] Full details of the definition and prognostic factors are provided in WHO Severe falciparum malaria. *Transactions of the Royal Society of Tropical Medicine and Hygiene*, 2000:94(Suppl. 1):1–90, and *Management of severe malaria: a practical handbook*, 2nd ed. Geneva, World Health Organization, 2000.

Management of severe malaria comprises four main areas: clinical assessment of the patient, specific antimalarial treatment, adjunctive therapy and supportive care.

8.3   Clinical assessment

Severe malaria is a medical emergency. The airway should be secured in unconscious patients and breathing and circulation assessed. The patient should be weighed or body weight estimated so that drugs, including antimalarials and fluids can be given on a body weight basis. An intravenous cannula should be inserted and immediate measurements of blood glucose (stick test), haematocrit/haemoglobin, parasitaemia and, in adults, renal function should be taken. A detailed clinical examination should be conducted, with particular note of the level of consciousness and record of the coma score. Several coma scores have been advocated. The Glasgow coma scale is suitable for adults, and the simple Blantyre modification or children's Glasgow coma scale are easily performed in children. Unconscious patients should have a lumbar puncture for cerebrospinal fluid analysis to exclude bacterial meningitis.

The degree of acidosis is an important determinant of outcome; the plasma bicarbonate or venous lactate level should therefore be measured if possible. If facilities are available, arterial or capillary blood pH and gases should be measured in patients who are unconscious, hyperventilating or in shock. Blood should be taken for cross-match, and (if possible) full blood count, platelet count, clotting studies, blood culture and full biochemistry should be conducted. The assessment of fluid balance is critical in severe malaria. Respiratory distress, in particular with acidotic breathing in severely anaemic children, often indicates hypovolaemia and requires prompt rehydration and, where indicated, blood transfusion (see also section 8.10.3).

8.4   Specific antimalarial treatment

It is essential that antimalarial treatment in full doses is given as soon as possible in severe malaria. Two classes of drugs are currently available for the parenteral treatment of severe malaria: the cinchona alkaloids (quinine and quinidine) and the artemisinin derivatives (artesunate, artemether and artemotil). Although there are a few areas where chloroquine is still effective, parenteral chloroquine is no longer recommended for the treatment of severe malaria because of widespread resistance. Intramuscular sulfadoxine–pyrimethamine is also not recommended.

8.4.1 Quinine

Quinine treatment for severe malaria was established before modern trial methods were developed. Several salts of quinine have been formulated for parenteral use, but the dihydrochloride is the most widely used. Peak concentrations following intramuscular quinine in severe malaria are similar to those following intravenous infusion. Pharmacokinetic modelling studies suggest that a loading dose of quinine of twice the maintenance dose (i.e. 20 mg salt/kg bw) reduces the time to reach therapeutic plasma concentrations. After the first day of treatment, the total daily maintenance dose of quinine is 30 mg salt/kg bw (usually divided into three equal administrations at 8 h intervals).

EVIDENCE: trials on dosage and route of administration of quinine[a]

Interventions: high first dose of quinine (loading dose 20 mg/kg bw) compared with non-loading dose regimen

> *Summary of RCTs:* a systematic review of two small trials showed shorter parasite and fever clearance time with high first-dose regimens but the trials were too small to show an impact on mortality.
>
> *Pharmacokinetic studies:* a 20 mg salt/kg bw loading dose results in effective blood levels of quinine being reached by the end of a 4-h infusion or within 4 h of i.m. administration. If a loading dose is not given, therapeutic concentrations may not be reached in the first 12 h of treatment.
>
> *Basis of decision:* pharmacokinetic studies.

Recommendation: use a loading dose of quinine of 20 mg salt/kg bw.

Interventions: quinine i.m. compared with quinine by i.v. infusion

> *Summary of RCTs:* one small trial of limited power did not demonstrate large differences.
>
> *Expert comment:* peak plasma concentrations are similar for both routes of administration. However, quinine i.m. may be erratically absorbed in severe malaria, particularly in patients with shock.
>
> *Basis of decision:* pharmacokinetic studies.

Recommendation: rate-controlled i.v. infusion is the preferred route of quinine administration, but if this cannot be given safely, then i.m. injection is a satisfactory alternative.

> **Interventions:** *quinine, rectal compared with quinine by i.m or i.v. infusion*
>
> > *Summary of RCTs:* one systematic review of 8 trials detected no difference in effect on parasites, clinical illness between the rectal group and either i.m or i.v. groups. Some studies however excluded patients with severe malaria.
> >
> > *Expert comment:* quinine dihydrochloride is locally irritant, quinine gluconate is less irritant.
> >
> > *Basis of decision:* systematic review.
>
> **Recommendation:** there is insufficient evidence to recommend rectal administration of quinine unless parenteral administration is not possible and no other effective options are available.

[a] See also Annex 9.1–9.3.

8.4.2 Artemisinin derivatives

Various artemisinin derivatives have been used in the treatment of severe malaria including artemether, artemisinin (rectal), artemotil and artesunate. The pharmacokinetic properties of artesunate are superior to those of artemether and artemotil as it is water soluble and can be given either by intravenous or intramuscular injection. Randomised trials comparing artesunate and quinine from South-East Asia show clear evidence of benefit with artesunate. In the largest multi-centre trial, which enrolled 1461 patients (including 202 children <15 years old), mortality was reduced by 34.7% compared to the quinine group. The results of this and smaller trials are consistent and suggest that artesunate is the treatment of choice for adults with severe malaria.

There are, however, still insufficient data for children, particularly from high transmission settings to make the same conclusion. An individual patient data meta-analysis of trials comparing artemether and quinine showed no difference in mortality in African children.

Although artesunate has better pharmacokinetic properties than artemether or artemotil, there are relatively few published comparative clinical trials. Concerns have been raised, regarding the possibility that the intrinsic benefits of artemether as an antimalarial may have been negated by its erratic absorption following intramuscular injection. Artemotil is very similar to artemether, but very few trials have been conducted.

EVIDENCE: trials of treatment of severe malaria with artemisinin derivatives compared to quinine[a]

Interventions: AS i.v. compared with quinine i.v. infusion

> *Summary of RCTs:* multi-centre trials enrolling 1461 patients, with mortality in the AS vs QN being 15% vs 22%. There was a relative reduction in mortality of 34.7% (95% CI: 18.5–47.6%; p = 0.002) in the AS group. QN was associated with hypoglycaemia (RR: 3.2, p = 0.009). Clear evidence of mortality benefit with artesunate.

> *Expert comment:* trials mainly in Asian adults, more information needed in children in higher transmission settings. There are no RCTs comparing AS with artemether i.m.

> *Basis of decision:* RCT

Recommendation: AS is the recommended first choice in areas of low-malaria transmission.

Interventions: artemether i.m. compared with quinine i.v. infusion

> *Summary of RCTs:* systematic review of 11 RCTs; analysis across all trials showed lower mortality with artemether, but this was not significant in an analysis of adequately concealed trials (RR: 0.8; 95% CI: 0.52–1.25). Within these, in an individual patient data analysis of 1919 adults and children, the odds ratio for deaths in artemether recipients was 0.8 (95% CI: 0.62–1.02). In the prospectively defined subgroup analysis of adults with multisystem failure, there was a significant difference in mortality in favour of artemether.

> *Expert comment:* artemether i.m. is erratically absorbed in severe malaria particularly in patients with shock.

> *Basis of decision:* systematic review.

Recommendation: artemether i.m. is an acceptable alternative to quinine i.v. infusion.

Interventions: artemotil i.m. compared with quinine by i.v. infusion

> *Summary of RCTs:* systematic review of two trials; the trials had insufficient power to show a difference.

> *Expert comment:* insufficient clinical trials and pharmacokinetic data to warrant a recommendation.

> *Basis of decision:* systematic review.

Recommendation: do not use artemotil unless alternatives are not available.

> *Interventions:* **artemisinin derivatives, rectal, compared with quinine by i.v. infusion**
>
>> *Summary of RCTs:* systematic review of three trials; the trials had insufficient power to show a difference.
>>
>> However, rectal artesunate has superior effect in reducing parasite densities compared to quinine (i.v. or i.m.) at 12 and 24 hours after administration.
>>
>> *Expert comment:* pharmacokinetic studies suggest highly variable but adequate absorption of rectal artemisinin and rectal artesunate. Rectal formulations have been developed for pre-referral use.
>>
>> *Basis of decision:* systematic review.
>
> **Recommendation:** use artemisinins rectally for complete treatment only when parenteral antimalarial treatment is not possible.
>
> [a] See also Annex 9.4–9.7.

8.4.3   Quinidine

Quinidine commonly causes hypotension and concentration-dependent prolongation of ventricular repolarization (QT prolongation). Quinidine is thus considered more toxic than quinine and should only be used if none of the other effective parenteral drugs are available. Electrocardiographic monitoring and frequent assessment of vital signs are required if quinidine is used.

Summary of recommendations on the treatment of severe malaria

RECOMMENDATIONS	LEVEL OF EVIDENCE
Severe malaria is a medical emergency.	E
After rapid clinical assessment and confirmation of the diagnosis, full doses of parenteral antimalarial treatment should be started without delay with whichever effective antimalarial is first available.	
Artesunate 2.4 mg/kg bw i.v. or i.m. given on admission (time = 0), then at 12 h and 24 h, then once a day is the recommended choice in low transmission areas or outside malaria endemic areas	S
For children in high transmission areas, the following antimalarial medicines are recommended as there is insufficient evidence to recommend any of these antimalarial medicines over another for severe malaria: – artesunate 2.4 mg/kg bw i.v. or i.m. given on admission (time = 0), then at 12 h and 24 h, then once a day; – artemether 3.2 mg/kg bw i.m. given on admission then 1.6 mg/kg bw per day; – quinine 20 mg salt/kg bw on admission (i.v. infusion or divided i.m. injection), then 10 mg/kg bw every 8 h; infusion rate should not exceed 5 mg salt/kg bw per hour.	S, T, O, E

8.5 Practical aspects of treatment

8.5.1 Artemisinins

Artemisinin is formulated as a suppository for rectal administration. Artemether and artemotil are formulated in oil and are given by intramuscular injection. They are both absorbed erratically, particularly in very severely ill patients. Artesunate is soluble in water and can be given either by intravenous or intramuscular injection. There are also rectal formulations of artesunate, artemether and dihydroartemisinin.

The dosing of artemisinin derivatives has been largely empirical. The doses recommended here are those that have been most widely studied. The only recent change is the higher maintenance dose of parenteral artesunate recommended (2.4 mg/kg bw), which is based on pharmacokinetic and pharmacodynamic studies and by extrapolation from studies with oral artesunate. Expert opinion is that the previously recommended maintenance dose of 1.2 mg/kg bw may have been insufficient in some patients.

Artesunate is dispensed as a powder of artesunic acid. This is dissolved in sodium bicarbonate (5%) to form sodium artesunate. The solution is then diluted in approximately 5 ml of 5% dextrose and given by intravenous injection or by intramuscular injection to the anterior thigh. The solution should be prepared freshly for each administration and should not be stored.

Artemether and artemotil are dispensed dissolved in oil (groundnut, sesame seed) and given by i.m. injection into the anterior thigh.

8.5.2 Quinine

Whereas many antimalarials are prescribed in terms of base, for historical reasons quinine doses are often recommended in terms of salt (usually sulfate for oral use and dihydrochloride for parenteral use). Recommendations for doses of this and other antimalarials should state clearly whether the salt or base is being referred to (doses with different salts must have the same base equivalents). Quinine must never be given by intravenous injection, as lethal hypotension may result. Quinine dihydrochloride should be given by rate-controlled infusion in saline or dextrose solutions at a rate not exceeding 5 mg salt/kg bw per hour. If this is not possible then it should be given by intramuscular injection to the anterior thigh, not the buttock (to avoid sciatic nerve injury). The first dose should be split, 10 mg/kg bw to each thigh. Undiluted quinine dihydrochloride at a concentration of 300 mg/ml is acidic (pH 2) and painful when given by intramuscular injection, so it is best either formulated or diluted to concentrations of 60–100 mg/ml for intramuscular injection. Gluconate salts are less acidic and better tolerated than the dihydrochloride salt when given by the intramuscular and rectal routes.

As the first dose (loading dose) is the most important in the treatment of severe malaria, this should be reduced only if there is clear evidence of adequate pre-treatment before presentation. Although quinine can cause hypotension if administered rapidly, and overdose is associated with blindness and deafness, these adverse effects are rare in the treatment of severe malaria. The dangers of insufficient treatment (i.e. death from malaria) exceed those from excessive treatment initially. After the second day of parenteral treatment, if there is no clinical improvement or in acute renal failure, the maintenance doses of quinine given by infusion should be reduced by one-third to avoid accumulation.

8.5.3 Adjustment of dosing in renal failure or hepatic dysfunction

The dosage of artemisinin derivatives does not need adjustment in vital organ dysfunction. Quinine (and quinidine) levels may accumulate in severe vital organ dysfunction. If there is no clinical improvement or the patient remains in acute renal failure the dose should be reduced by one-third after 48 h. Dosage adjustments are not necessary if patients are receiving either haemodialysis or haemofiltration. Dosage adjustment by one-third is necessary in patients with hepatic dysfunction.

8.6   Follow-on treatment

Following initial parenteral treatment, once the patient can tolerate oral therapy, it is essential to continue and complete treatment with an effective oral anti-malarial. Current practice is to continue the same medicine orally as given parenterally to complete a full 7 days of treatment. In non-pregnant adults, doxycycline is added to either quinine, artesunate or artemether and should also be given for 7 days. Doxycycline is preferred to other tetracyclines because it can be given once daily, and does not accumulate in renal failure. But as treatment with doxycycline only starts when the patient has recovered sufficiently, the doxycycline course finishes after the quinine, artemether or artesunate course. Where available, clindamycin may be substituted in children and pregnant women, as doxycycline cannot be given to these groups. Although following parenteral treatment with a full course of oral ACT (artesunate + amodiaquine or artemether-lumefantrine) is theoretically a good alternative, this has not been evaluated in clinical trials.

The recommendation from experts' opinion is to complete treatment in severe malaria following parenteral drug administration by giving a full course of combination therapy, ACT or quinine + clindamycin or doxycycline. Regimens containing mefloquine should be avoided if the patient presented initially with impaired consciousness. This is because of an increased incidence of neuropsychiatric complications associated with mefloquine following cerebral malaria.

8.7   Pre-referral treatment options[16]

The risk of death from severe malaria is greatest in the first 24 h, yet in most malaria endemic countries, the transit time between referral and arrival at appropriate health facilities is usually prolonged thus delaying the commencement of appropriate antimalarial treatment, during which time the patient may deteriorate or die. It is recommended that patients are treated with the first dose of one of the recommended treatments by the parenteral route if possible or by the intra-rectal route before referral (unless the referral time is very short). This could be intramuscular artemether, artesunate or quinine, or a rectal formulation of artemisinin or artesunate.

Summary of recommendations on pre-referral treatment for severe falciparum malaria

RECOMMENDATIONS	LEVEL OF EVIDENCE
The following may be given:	
– artesunate or artemisinin by rectal administration	T, E
– artesunate or artemether i.m.	E
– quinine i.m.	O, E

8.7.1   Pre-referral and continued treatment with rectal artemisinins

The administration of an artemisinin by the rectal route as pre-referral treatment is feasible even at the community level.

There is insufficient evidence to show whether rectal artesunate is as good as intravenous or intramuscular options in the management of severe malaria. The recommendation, therefore, is to use artesunate or artemisinin suppositories only as pre-referral treatment and to refer the patient to a facility where complete parenteral treatment with artesunate, quinine or artemether

---

[16] Further infromation is provided in Annex 9.8

can be instituted. If, however, referral is impossible, rectal treatment should be continued until the patient can tolerate oral medication, at which point a full course of the recommended ACT for uncomplicated malaria in the locality can be administered.

8.7.2 Dosing for antimalarials given by suppository

Artemisinin derivatives

Artemisinin suppositories are not widely available. Doses used have been variable and empiric: 10–40 mg/kg bw (at 0, 4 or 12, 24, 48 and 72 h). Some studies have given a maintenance dose of one- to two-thirds of the initial dose. Artesunate suppositories* are given in a dose of 10 mg/kg bw daily. The individual suppositories contain either 50, 100 or 400 mg of artesunate. Recommendations for artesunate suppositories for pre-referral treatment of severe malaria are provided in Tables 5 and 6.

Initial (pre-referral) treatment with rectal artesunate

The appropriate single dose of artesunate given by suppository should be administered rectally as soon as the presumptive diagnosis of severe malaria is made. In the event that an artesunate suppository is expelled from the rectum within 30 min of insertion, a second suppository should be inserted and, especially in young children, the buttocks should be held together, for 10 min to ensure retention of the rectal dose of artesunate.

For adults: one or more artesunate suppositories inserted in the rectum, dose as indicated in Table 5. The dose should be given once and followed as soon as possible by definitive therapy for malaria.

Table 5. **Dosage* for initial (pre-referral) treatment in adult patients (aged ≥16 years)**

Weight (kg)	Artesunate dose	Regimen (single dose)
<40	10 mg/kg bw	Use appropriate no. of 100-mg rectal suppositories (see Table 6)
40–59	400 mg	One 400-mg suppository
60–80	800 mg	Two 400-mg suppositories
>80	1200 mg	Three 400-mg suppositories

* It should be noted that the clinical trial data with rectal artesunate relate to a single suppository formulation and presentation[17] which has well characterized absorption kinetics and so cannot necessarily be extrapolated to other rectal formulations of artesunate.

---

[17] This product is being developed by the UNDP/UNICEF/World Bank/WHO Special Programme for Research and Training in Tropical Diseases.

For children: one or more artesunate suppositories inserted in the rectum as indicated in Table 6. The dose should be given once and followed as soon as possible by definitive therapy for malaria.

Table 6. **Dosage for initial (pre-referral) treatment in children (aged 2–15 years) and weighing at least 5 kg**

Weight (kg)	Age	Artesunate dose (mg)	Regimen (single dose)
5–8.9	0–12 months	50	One 50-mg suppository
9–19	13–42 months	100	One 100-mg suppository
20–29	43–60 months	200	Two 100-mg suppositories
30–39	6–13 years	300	Three 100-mg suppositories
>40	>14 years	400	One 400-mg suppository

Quinine

The intrarectal dose used in treatment trials in Africa was either 12 mg/kg bw quinine base every 12 h without a loading dose, or 8 mg/kg bw every 8 h, also without a loading dose. The retention and absorption of quinine is dependent on pH. Results with gluconate salts (pH 4.5) cannot be extrapolated to more acidic solutions (such as the dihydrochloride salt, pH 2).

8.8 Adjunctive treatment

In an attempt to reduce the unacceptably high mortality of severe malaria, various adjunctive treatments for the complications of malaria have been evaluated in clinical trials. These are summarized in Table 7 and further information is given in sections 8.9 and 8.10.

Table 7. **Immediate clinical management of severe manifestations and complications of falciparum malaria**

Manifestation/complication	Immediate management[a]
Coma (cerebral malaria)	Maintain airway, place patient on his or her side, exclude other treatable causes of coma (e.g. hypoglycaemia, bacterial meningitis); avoid harmful ancillary treatment such as corticosteroids, heparin and adrenaline; intubate if necessary.
Hyperpyrexia	Administer tepid sponging, fanning, cooling blanket and antipyretic drugs.
Convulsions	Maintain airways; treat promptly with intravenous or rectal diazepam or intramuscular paraldehyde.
Hypoglycaemia (blood glucose concentration of <2.2 mmol/l; <40 mg/100ml)	Check blood glucose, correct hypoglycaemia and maintain with glucose-containing infusion.
Severe anaemia (haemoglobin <5 g/100ml or packed cell volume <15%)	Transfuse with screened fresh whole blood
Acute pulmonary oedema[b]	Prop patient up at an angle of 45°, give oxygen, give a diuretic, stop intravenous fluids, intubate and add positive end-expiratory pressure/continuous positive airway pressure in life-threatening hypoxaemia.
Acute renal failure	Exclude pre-renal causes, check fluid balance and urinary sodium; if in established renal failure add haemofiltration or haemodialysis, or if unavailable, peritoneal dialysis. The benefits of diuretics/dopamine in acute renal failure are not proven.
Spontaneous bleeding and coagulopathy	Transfuse with screened fresh whole blood (cryoprecipitate, fresh frozen plasma and platelets if available); give vitamin K injection.
Metabolic acidosis	Exclude or treat hypoglycaemia, hypovolaemia and septicaemia. If severe add haemofiltration or haemodialysis.
Shock	Suspect septicaemia, take blood for cultures; give parenteral antimicrobials, correct haemodynamic disturbances.
Hyperparasitaemia	See section 8.14.

[a] It is assumed that appropriate antimalarial treatment will have been started in all cases.

[b] Prevent by avoiding excess hydration.

8.9   Continuing supportive care

Patients with severe malaria require intensive nursing, in an intensive care unit if possible. Following the initial assessment and the start of antimalarial treatment, clinical observations should be made as frequently as possible. These should include recording of vital signs, with an accurate assessment of respiratory rate and pattern, coma score, and urine output. Blood glucose should be checked, using rapid stick tests every 4 h if possible, particularly in unconscious patients. Convulsions should be treated promptly with intravenous or rectal diazepam or intramuscular paraldehyde.

Fluid requirements should be assessed individually. Adults with severe malaria are very vulnerable to fluid overload and there is a thin dividing line between underhydration, and thus worsening renal impairment, and overhydration, with the risk of precipitating pulmonary oedema. If the patient becomes oliguric (< 0.4 ml of urine/kg bw per hour) despite adequate rehydration, and the blood urea or creatinine are rising or already high, then fluids should be restricted to replace insensible losses only. Children, on the other hand, are more likely to be dehydrated and may respond well to a bolus of fluid. The fluid regimen must also be tailored around infusion of the antimalarial drugs. Central venous pressure should be maintained at 0–5 cm. If the venous pressure is elevated (usually because of excessive fluid administration), the patient should be nursed with the head raised at an angle of 45° and, if necessary, intravenous furosemide should be given. If available, heamofiltration should be started early for acute renal failure or severe metabolic acidosis unresponsive to rehydration.

If blood glucose is < 2.2 mmol/l then hypoglycaemia should be treated immediately (0.3–0.5 g/kg bw of glucose). Hypoglycaemia should be suspected in any patient who deteriorates suddenly. Stick tests may overestimate the frequency of hypoglycaemia, so laboratory confirmation may be necessary.

Patients with acute pulmonary oedema should be nursed in an upright position and given oxygen, and filling pressures on the right side of the heart should be reduced with whichever treatments are available (loop diuretics, opiates, venodilators, venesection, haemofiltration, dialysis). The right-sided pressure should be reduced to the lowest level compatible with an adequate cardiac output. Positive pressure ventilation should be started (if available) early if the patient becomes hypoxic.

Fewer than 5% of patients with severe malaria develop clinically significant disseminated intravascular coagulation. These patients should be given fresh blood transfusions and vitamin K. Patients with secondary pneumonia should be given empirical treatment with a third-generation cephalosporin, unless admitted with clear evidence of aspiration, in which case penicillin or clindamycin is adequate. Children with persistent fever despite parasite clearance may have a systematic *Salmonella* infection, although in the majority of cases of persistent fever no other pathogen is identified after parasite clearance. Urinary tract infections are common in catheterized patients. Antibiotic treatments should take account of likely local antibiotic sensitivity patterns.

8.10 Additional aspects of clinical management

8.10.1 Diagnosis

The differential diagnosis of fever in a severely ill patient is broad. Coma and fever may result from meningoencephalitis or malaria. Cerebral malaria is not associated with signs of meningeal irritation (neck stiffness, photophobia, Kernig sign) but the patient may be opisthotonic. As untreated bacterial meningitis is almost invariably fatal, a diagnostic lumbar puncture should be performed to exclude this condition. There is also considerable clinical overlap between septicaemia, pneumonia and severe malaria – and these conditions may coexist. In malaria endemic areas particularly, where parasitaemia is common in the young age group, it is often impossible to rule out septicaemia in a shocked or severely ill obtunded child. Where possible, blood should always be taken on admission for culture, and if there is any doubt, empirical antibiotic treatment should be started immediately along with antimalarial treatment.

8.10.2 Other treatments

Many other supportive strategies and interventions have been proposed in severe malaria, but very few are supported by evidence of benefit, and many have proved harmful.

Heparin, prostacyclin, deferoxamine, pentoxifylline, low molecular weight dextran, urea, high-dose corticosteroids, acetylsalicylic acid, deferoxamine, anti-tumour necrosis factor antibody, cyclosporin, dichloroacetate, adrenaline and hyperimmune serum have all been suggested – but none of these is recommended. Evidence on use of corticosteroids is summarized in the box below.

EVIDENCE: **trials of routine use of corticosteroids (e.g. dexamethasone) in the treatment of severe falciparum malaria[a]**

Interventions: corticosteroids i.v.

> *Summary of RCTs:* one systematic review and no additional trials. No significant difference in mortality; increased risk of gastrointestinal bleeding.
>
> *Expert comment:* no additional information.
>
> *Basis of decision:* systematic review.

Recommendation: do not use corticosteroids.

---

[a] See also Annex 9.9.

Severe metabolic acidosis is common but apart from correction of hypovolaemia and anaemia, no specific treatment is of proven value. Significant electrolyte abnormalities are relatively unusual, and potassium supplementation is often not required in the acute phase. The optimum fluid resuscitation regimens, the thresholds for blood transfusion, the role of exchange transfusion, and the management of seizures remain areas of uncertainty, and these are discussed in more detail below. The optimum body positioning in comatose patients, and the timing and type of feeding in patients who remain unconscious for > 24 h have not been studied. It is generally agreed that early ventilation for respiratory abnormalities and early management of renal failure or severe metabolic acidosis are beneficial. In acute renal failure, haemofiltration is associated with a lower mortality, and more rapid correction of biochemical abnormalities compared with peritoneal dialysis. There have been no comparative trials of haemodialysis and haemofiltration.

8.10.3 Fluid therapy

Patients, especially children with severe malaria may be dehydrated. However, the degree of fluid depletion varies considerably. As a result, it is not possible to give general recommendations on fluid replacement. Each patient must be individually assessed and fluid resuscitation based on estimated deficit. In high-transmission settings where severe malaria is confined to childhood, children commonly present with severe anaemia and hyperventilation (sometimes termed "respiratory distress"). In the past this was ascribed to "anaemic heart failure" (i.e. pulmonary oedema), and sometimes diuretics were administered. It is now clear that this syndrome is not a result of anaemic heart failure, but results from severe metabolic acidosis and anaemia, and so should be treated by blood transfusion. In general children tolerate rapid fluid resuscitation better than adults, and are less likely to develop pulmonary oedema. In adults, there is a very thin dividing line between overhydration, which may produce pulmonary oedema, and underhydration contributing to shock and worsening acidosis and renal impairment. Careful and frequent evaluations of the jugular venous pressure, peripheral perfusion, venous filling, skin turgor and urine output should be made. Where there is uncertainty over the jugular venous pressure, and if nursing facilities permit, a central venous catheter should be inserted and the central venous pressure measured directly. The optimum rate of resuscitation, the role of colloids compared with crystalloids, and the optimum electrolyte composition of the replacement fluid have not been determined.

8.10.4 Blood transfusion

Severe malaria is associated with rapid development of anaemia as infected and uninfected erythrocytes are removed from the circulation. In areas of high stable transmission, severe anaemia in young children is the principal manifestation of severe falciparum malaria. Ideally fresh blood should be transfused, and the patient's relatives are often willing donors. However, in most settings cross-matched virus-free blood is in short supply. As with fluid resuscitation, there have not been enough studies to provide strong evidence-based recommendations, so the recommendations given here are based on expert opinion. In high-transmission settings, blood transfusion is recommended for children with a haemoglobin level of <5 g/100 ml (haematocrit <15%). Mortality as a direct result of anaemia rises at lower haemoglobin levels. In low-transmission settings, a threshold of 20% (haemoglobin 7 g/100ml) is recommended. These general recommendations still need to be tailored to the individual, as the pathological consequences of rapid development of anaemia are worse than those of acute on chronic anaemia, where there has been adaptation and a compensatory right shift in the oxygen dissociation curve (Annex 9.10).

8.10.5 Exchange blood transfusion (EBT)

There have been many anecdotal reports and several series claiming benefit for EBT in severe malaria but no comparative trials, and there is no consensus on whether it reduces mortality or how it might work. The rationale for EBT has been variously proposed as:

- removing infected red blood cells from the circulation and therefore lowering the parasite burden (although only the circulating relatively non-pathogenic stages are removed – and this is also achieved rapidly with artemisinin derivatives);
- reducing rapidly both the antigen load and the burden of parasite-derived toxins, metabolites and toxic mediators produced by the host;
- replacing the rigid unparasitized red cells by more deformable cells and therefore alleviating microcirculatory obstruction.

EBT requires intensive nursing and a relatively large volume of blood, and carries significant risks. There is no consensus on the indications, benefits and dangers involved, or on practical details such as the volume of blood that should be exchanged. It is therefore not possible to make any recommendation regarding the use of EBT.

8.10.6 Use of anticonvulsants

Seizures are common in cerebral malaria, particularly in children. The treatment of convulsions in cerebral malaria with intravenous (or, if not possible, rectal) benzodiazepines or intramuscular paraldehyde is similar to that for repeated seizures from any cause. In a large double-blind placebo-controlled evaluation of a single intramuscular injection of 20 mg/kg bw of phenobarbital (phenobarbitone) in children with cerebral malaria there was a reduction in seizures but a significant increase in mortality in phenobarbital recipients. This resulted from respiratory arrest, and was associated with additional benzodiazepine use. Clearly the 20 mg/kg dose of phenobarbital should not be given without respiratory support, but it is not known, whether a lower dose would be effective and safer or whether, if ventilation is given, mortality would not be increased. In the absence of further information, prophylactic anticonvulsants are not recommended.

> **EVIDENCE: trials on use of phenobarbital for the treatment of convulsions in severe falciparum malaria[a]**
>
> *Interventions: phenobarbital i.v.*
>
> > *Summary of RCTs:* systematic review of three trials. In the two trials with adequate blinding, death was more common with phenobarbital.
> >
> > *Expert comment:* no additional information.
> >
> > *Basis of decision:* systematic review.
>
> Recommendation: avoid routine use of phenobarbital.

[a] See also Annex 9.11.

8.10.7 Concomitant use of antibiotics

The threshold for administering antibiotic treatment should be low in severe malaria. Septicaemia and severe malaria are associated and there is diagnostic overlap, particularly in children. Unexplained deterioration may result from a supervening bacterial infection. Although enteric bacteria (notably *Salmonella*) have predominated in most trial series, a variety of bacteria have been cultured from the blood of patients diagnosed as having severe malaria, and so broad-spectrum antibiotic treatment should be given initially.

8.11   Treatment during pregnancy

Pregnant women, particularly in the second and third trimesters of pregnancy are more likely to develop severe malaria than other adults, often complicated by pulmonary oedema and hypoglycaemia. Maternal mortality is approximately 50%, which is higher than in non-pregnant adults. Fetal death and premature labour are common. The role of early Caesarean section for the viable live fetus is unproven, but is recommended by many authorities. Obstetric advice should be sought at an early stage, the paediatricians alerted, and blood glucose checked frequently. Hypoglycaemia should be expected and is often recurrent if the patient is receiving quinine. Antimalarials should be given in full doses. Severe malaria may also present immediately following delivery. Postpartum bacterial infection is a common complication in these cases. Falciparum malaria has also been associated with severe mid-trimester haemolytic anaemia in Nigeria. This often requires transfusion, in addition to antimalarial treatment and folate supplementation.

Parenteral antimalarials should be given to pregnant women with severe malaria in full doses without delay. Artesunate or artemether are preferred over quinine in the second and third trimesters because quinine is associated with recurrent hypoglycaemia. Recent evidence shows that in non pregnant adults with severe malaria in areas of low transmission, artesunate was superior to quinine, reducing mortality by 35% compared to quinine, which makes artesunate the preferred option in the second and third trimesters. In the first trimester, the risk of hypoglycaemia associated with quinine is lower, and the uncertainties over the safety of the artemisinin derivatives are greater. However, weighing these risks against the above evidence in favour of the efficacy of artesunate, and until more evidence becomes available, both artesunate and quinine may be considered as options. Treatment must not be delayed so if only one of the drugs artesunate, artemether or quinine is available it should be started immediately.

EVIDENCE: treatment for severe falciparum malaria in pregnant women

Interventions: AS, artemether, quinine (all parenteral)

Summary of RCTs: none.

Expert comment: complications of severe malaria are more frequent in pregnant women than in non-pregnant adults. Artesunate reduces the mortality of severe malaria in non pregnant adults compared with quinine in low transmission situations. The artemisinin derivatives (artesunate and artemether) may also have safety advantages compared with quinine in the second and third trimesters of pregnancy because they do not cause recurrent hypoglycaemia. In the first trimester, the risk of hypoglycaemia associated with quinine is lower, and the uncertainties over the safety of the artemisinin derivatives are greater.

Basis of decision: expert opinion.

Recommendation: use the parenteral antimalarial treatment locally available for severe malaria in full doses. Where available, AS is the first, and artemether the second option in the second and third trimesters.

In the first trimester, until more evidence becomes available, both artesunate and quinine may be considered as options.

8.12   Management in epidemic situations

Management of severe falciparum malaria in epidemic situations will often take place in temporary clinics or in situations in which staff shortages and high workloads make intensive care monitoring difficult. Drug treatment should therefore be as simple and safe as possible, with simple dosing schedules and a minimum need for monitoring. Artesunate has been shown to reduce mortality of severe malaria, but with the current artesunate formulation, drawing the drug into a syringe takes two dissolution-dilution steps. In some circumstances this may not be possible. Parenteral quinine requires either intravenous infusions or a three times a day intramuscular regimen, plus monitoring of blood glucose. Thus the simple once a day regimens and the ease of drawing up and administering intramuscular artemether make this a suitable alternative for severe malaria in most epidemic situations. Experience with artesunate suppositories in epidemic situations is limited. Their use may be appropriate in severely ill patients who are unable to swallow oral medication when intramuscular artemether (or quinine by intravenous infusion) is unavailable. If artesunate suppositories are used, patients should be moved as soon as possible to a facility where intramuscular or intravenous therapy can be started.

When the patient cannot be moved, continued treatment with rectal artesunate is appropriate until oral drugs can be taken. It is essential that a full course of antimalarial treatment is completed.

8.12.1 Treatment during pregnancy in epidemic situations

In epidemic settings where the need for simplicity is paramount, intramuscular artemether is the drug of choice for severe malaria in all trimesters of pregnancy.

Summary of recommendation on treatment of severe falciparum malaria in pregnant women in epidemic situations

RECOMMENDATION	LEVEL OF EVIDENCE
Artesunate by the intravenous route is the treatment of choice, but if not possible, artemether by the intramuscular route is the preferred alternative for severe malaria in pregnancy during a malaria epidemic.	E

8.13 Hyperparasitaemia[18]

Patients with high parasite counts are known to be at increased risk of dying, although the relationship between parasite counts and prognosis varies at different levels of malaria endemicity. Many hyperparasitaemic patients have evidence of vital organ dysfunction but there is a large subgroup in which no other manifestations of severe disease are present. These patients have symptoms and signs compatible with a diagnosis of uncomplicated malaria in association with a high parasite count (sometimes termed uncomplicated hyperparasitaemia). The relevance for treatment is firstly the increased risk of progressing to severe malaria, and secondly the generally higher treatment failure rates. This is of particular concern as resistance to antimalarials is most likely to arise in patients with heavy parasite burdens and little or no immunity. In a low-transmission area in north-west Thailand, the overall mortality of uncomplicated falciparum malaria was 0.1%, but in patients with parasitaemia of >4% it was 3%. In areas of moderate or high transmission, much higher parasitaemias are often well tolerated, however. There is not enough evidence to provide a firm recommendation on the definition of hyperparasitaemia, although ≥5% parasitaemia in a low-transmission setting and ≥10% in a higher transmission setting are commonly used.

---

[18] Further information is provided in Annex 9.12

8.13.1 Treatment of hyperparasitaemia

Available evidence indicates that use of oral treatment under close supervision is effective in the treatment of patients with hyperparasitaemia who have no other features of severe malaria. Parenteral treatment should, however, be substituted at any time if there is concern. The rapidity of action of the artemisinin derivatives makes them ideal drugs. The standard treatment course should be given, as there is insufficient information on the safety of higher doses of the partner drug. Alternatively, the first dose of artemisinin derivative can be given parenterally or rectally to ensure adequate absorption, followed by a full course of ACT. Mefloquine-containing regimens in which the tablets are dispensed separately should be given such that mefloquine is given on days 2 and 3, rather than day 1, when it is better tolerated, with a lower incidence of early vomiting.

The optimum duration of treatment for hyperparasitaemia is still unresolved. Data to support the suggestion that patients should be treated conservatively with 7 days of an artemisinin derivative, plus a full course of partner medicine (e.g. artesunate 7 days + mefloquine 25 mg/kg bw divided over 2 days) are lacking. A longer ACT course than is recommended for uncomplicated malaria may not be possible in places where only fixed-dose combinations are available.

Summary of recommendations on the treatment of hyperparasitaemia in falciparum malaria

RECOMMENDATIONS	LEVEL OF EVIDENCE
Hyperparasitaemic patients with no other signs of severe disease should be treated with oral artemisinin derivatives under the following conditions:	O, E
– patients must be monitored closely for the first 48 h after the start of treatment,	
– if the patient does not retain oral medication, parenteral treatment should be given without delay.	
Non-immune patients with parasitaemia of > 20% should receive parenteral antimalarial treatment.	E

9. TREATMENT OF MALARIA CAUSED BY *P. VIVAX*, *P. OVALE* OR *P. MALARIAE* [19]

P. vivax, the second most important species causing human malaria, accounts for about 40% of malaria cases worldwide and is the dominant malaria species outside Africa. It is prevalent in endemic areas in the Middle East, Asia, Oceania and Central and South America. In Africa, it is rare except in the Horn and it is almost absent in West Africa. In most areas where *P. vivax* is prevalent, malaria transmission rates are low, and the affected populations therefore achieve little immunity to this parasite. Consequently, people of all ages are at risk. The other two human malaria parasite species *P. malariae* and *P. ovale* are generally less prevalent but are distributed worldwide especially in the tropical areas of Africa.

Among the four species of *Plasmodium* that affect humans, only *P. vivax* and *P. ovale* form hypnozoites, parasite stages in the liver that can result in multiple relapses of infection, weeks to months after the primary infection. Thus a single infection causes repeated bouts of illness. This affects the development and schooling of children and debilitates adults, thereby impairing human and economic development in affected populations. The objective of treating malaria caused by *P. vivax* and *P. ovale* is to cure both the blood stage and the liver stage infections, and thereby prevent both relapse and recrudescence. This is called radical cure. Infection with *P. vivax* during pregnancy, as with *P. falciparum*, reduces birth weight. In primigravidae, the reduction is approximately two-thirds of that associated with *P. falciparum* (110 g compared to 170 g), but this adverse effect does not decline with successive pregnancies as with *P. falciparum* infections. Indeed, in the one large series in which this was studied, it increased. Reduction in birth weight ($<$ 2500 g) increases the risk of neonatal death.

9.1 Diagnosis

The clinical features of uncomplicated malaria are too non-specific for a clinical diagnosis of the species of malaria infection to be made. Diagnosis of *P. vivax* malaria is based on microscopy. Although rapid diagnostic tests based on immunochromatographic methods are available for the detection of non-falciparum malaria, their sensitivities below parasite densities of 500/µl are low. Their relatively high cost is a further impediment to their wide use in endemic areas. Molecular markers for genotyping *P. vivax* parasites have been developed to assist epidemiological and treatment studies but these are still under evaluation.

---

[19] Further information is provided in Annex 10.

9.2 Susceptibility of *P. vivax, P. ovale* and *P. malariae* to antimalarials

There are very few recent data on the *in vivo* susceptibility of *P. ovale* and *P. malariae* to antimalarials. Both species are regarded as very sensitive to chloroquine, although there is a single recent report of chloroquine resistance in *P. malariae*. Experience indicates that *P. ovale* and *P. malariae* are also susceptible to amodiaquine, mefloquine and the artemisinin derivatives. Their susceptibility to antifolate antimalarials such as sulfadoxine-pyrimethamine is less certain. *P. vivax* susceptibility has been studied extensively, and now that short-term culture methodologies have been standardized, clinical studies have been supported by *in vitro* observations. *P. vivax* is still generally very sensitive to chloroquine, although resistance is prevalent and increasing in some areas, notably Oceania, Indonesia and Peru (see Annex A.6.4). Resistance to pyrimethamine has increased rapidly in some areas, and sulfadoxine-pyrimethamine is consequently ineffective. There are insufficient data on current susceptibility to proguanil and chlorproguanil, although resistance to proguanil was selected rapidly when it was first used in *P.vivax* endemic areas. In general, *P. vivax* is sensitive to all the other antimalarial drugs; it is more sensitive than *P. falciparum* to the artemisinin derivatives, and slightly less sensitive to mefloquine (although mefloquine is still effective). In contrast to *P. falciparum*, asexual stages of *P. vivax* are susceptible to primaquine. Thus chloroquine + primaquine can be considered as a combination treatment. The only drugs with significant activity against the hypnozoites are the 8-amino-quinolines (bulaquine, primaquine, tafenoquine). There is no standardized in vitro method of drug assessment for hypnozoiticidal activity. *In vivo* assessment suggests that tolerance of *P. vivax* to primaquine in East Asia and Oceania is greater than elsewhere.

9.3 Treatment of uncomplicated vivax malaria

9.3.1 Blood stage infection

There have been fewer studies on the treatment of malaria caused by *P. vivax* than of falciparum malaria – only 11% of 435 published before 2004. For chloroquine-sensitive vivax malaria (i.e. in most places where *P. vivax* is prevalent) the conventional oral chloroquine dose of 25 mg base/kg bw is well tolerated and effective. Some have advocated lower total doses, but this is not recommended as it might encourage the emergence of resistance. Chloroquine is given in an initial dose of 10 mg base/kg bw followed by either 5 mg/kg bw at 6 h, 24 h and 48 h or, more commonly, by 10 mg/kg bw on the second day and 5 mg/kg bw on the third day. It is also clear that if ACT treatment is given, the response is as good as or better than in falciparum malaria. The exception to this is a regimen containing sulfadoxine-pyrimethamine. It appears that *P. vivax* has developed resistance to sulfadoxine-pyrimethamine more rapidly than has *P. falciparum,* so that artesunate + sulfadoxine-pyrimethamine may not be effective against *P. vivax* in many areas.

Chloroquine-resistant vivax malaria

There are relatively few data on treatment responses in chloroquine-resistant vivax malaria. Studies from Indonesia indicate that amodiaquine is efficacious, and there is some evidence that mefloquine and quinine can also be used. The artemisinin derivatives would also be expected to be highly effective, and artemether-lumefantrine could be an alternative treatment. However, there are insufficient clinical data to confirm this.

9.3.2   Liver stage infection

To achieve radical cure, relapses must be prevented by giving primaquine. The frequency and pattern of relapses varies geographically, however. It has become clear in recent years that whereas 50–60% of *P. vivax* infections in South-East Asia relapse, the frequency is lower in Indonesia (30%) and the Indian subcontinent (15–20%). Some *P. vivax* infections in the Korean peninsula (now the most northerly of human malarias) have an incubation period of nearly one year. Thus the preventive efficacy of primaquine must be set against the prevalent relapse frequency. It appears that the total dose of 8-aminoquinoline given is the main determinant of curative efficacy against liver-stage infection. There is no evidence that the short courses of primaquine widely recommended (such as 5-day regimens) have any efficacy. Primaquine should be given for 14 days. The usual adult oral dose is 15 mg base (0.25 mg/kg bw per day) but in South-East Asia, particularly Indonesia, and in Oceania, higher doses (0.5 mg base/kg bw per day) are required. Primaquine causes abdominal discomfort when taken on an empty stomach; it should always be taken with food.

There has been debate as to whether primaquine should be given in endemic areas. Repeated vivax malaria relapses are debilitating at any age, but if reinfection is very frequent, then the risks of widespread use of primaquine may exceed the benefits. In low-transmission areas, the benefits of deploying primaquine are considered to exceed the risks, but in areas of sustained high transmission (such as on the island of New Guinea), *P. vivax* infection is very frequent, immunity is acquired, and the risks of widespread deployment of primaquine are considered to outweigh the benefits.

Primaquine and glucose-6-phosphate dehydrogenase deficiency

The inherited sex-linked deficiency in glucose-6-phosphate dehydrogenase (G6PD) is associated with some protection against falciparum malaria, but increased susceptibility to oxidant haemolysis. The prevalence of G6PD deficiency varies but can be as high as 30%. There are many different genotypes, each with different levels of deficiency. Primaquine is an oxidant and causes variable haemolysis in G6PD-deficient individuals. Fortunately primaquine is eliminated rapidly and so haemolysis is self-limiting provided no further medicine is taken. Screening for G6PD deficiency is not generally available outside hospitals, although rapid tests are under development. Many patients are therefore unaware of their G6PD status. If a patient is known to be severely G6PD deficient then primaquine should not be given. For the majority of patients with mild variants of the deficiency, primaquine should be given in a dose of 0.75 mg base/kg bw once a week for 8 weeks. If significant haemolysis occurs on treatment then primaquine should be stopped.

Summary of recommendations on the treatment of uncomplicated vivax malaria

RECOMMENDATIONS	LEVEL OF EVIDENCE
Chloroquine 25 mg base/kg bw divided over 3 days, combined with primaquine 0.25 mg base/kg bw, taken with food once daily for 14 days is the treatment of choice for chloroquine-sensitive infections. In Oceania and South-East Asia the dose of primaquine should be 0.5 mg/kg bw.	O, E
Amodiaquine (30 mg base/kg bw divided over 3 days as 10 mg/kg bw single daily doses) combined with primaquine should be given for chloroquine-resistant vivax malaria.	O, E
In moderate G6PD deficiency, primaquine 0.75 mg base/kg bw should be given once a week for 8 weeks. In severe G6PD deficiency, primaquine should not be given.	O, E
Where ACT has been adopted as the first-line treatment for *P. falciparum* malaria, it may also be used for *P. vivax* malaria in combination with primaquine for radical cure. Artesunate + sulfadoxine-pyrimethamine is the exception as it will not be effective against *P. vivax* in many places.	O, E

9.4 Treatment of severe vivax malaria

Although *P. vivax* malaria is considered to be a benign malaria, with a very low case-fatality ratio, it may still cause a severe and debilitating febrile illness. It can also very occasionally result in severe disease as in falciparum malaria. Severe vivax malaria manifestations that have been reported are cerebral malaria, severe anaemia, severe thrombocytopenia and pancytopenia, jaundice, spleen rupture, acute renal failure and acute respiratory distress syndrome. Severe anaemia and acute pulmonary oedema are not uncommon. The underlying mechanisms of severe manifestations are not well understood.

Prompt and effective treatment and case management should be the same as for severe and complicated falciparum malaria (see section 8).

9.5 Treatment of malaria caused by *P. ovale* and *P. malariae*

Resistance of *P. ovale* and *P. malariae* to antimalarials is not well characterized and infections caused by these two species are considered to be generally sensitive to chloroquine. Only one study, conducted in Indonesia, has reported resistance to chloroquine in *P. malariae*. The recommended treatment for the relapsing malaria caused by *P. ovale* is the same as that given to achieve radical cure in vivax malaria, i.e. with chloroquine and primaquine. *P. malariae* should be treated with the standard regimen of chloroquine as for vivax malaria, but it does not require radical cure with primaquine as no hypnozoites are formed in infection with this species.

P.ovale mainly occurs in areas of high stable transmission where the risk of re-infection is high. In such settings, primaquine treatment is not indicated.

9.6 Monitoring therapeutic efficacy for vivax malaria

The antimalarial sensitivity of vivax malaria needs monitoring, to track and respond to emerging resistance to chloroquine. The 28-day *in vivo* test for *P. vivax* is similar to that for *P. falciparum* (see Annex 6), although the interpretation is slightly different. Genotyping may distinguish a reinfection from a recrudescence and from acquisition of a new infection, but it is not possible to distinguish reliably between a relapse and a recrudescence as they derive from the same infection. If parasitaemia recurs within 16 days of administering treatment then relapse is unlikely, but after that time, relapse cannot be distinguished from a recrudescence. Any *P. vivax* infection that recurs within 28 days, whatever its origin, must be resistant to chloroquine (or any other slowly eliminated antimalarial) provided adequate treatment has been given. In the case of chloroquine, adequate absorption can be confirmed by measurement of the whole blood concentration at the time of recurrence. Any *P. vivax* infection that has grown *in vivo* through a chloroquine blood concentration ≥100 ng/ml must be chloroquine resistant. Short-term *in vitro* culture allows assessment of *in vitro* susceptibility. There are no molecular markers yet identified for chloroquine resistance. Antifolate resistance can be monitored by molecular genotyping of the gene that encodes dihydrofolate reductase (*Pvdhfr*).

10. MIXED MALARIA INFECTIONS

Mixed malaria infections are common. In Thailand, despite low levels of malaria transmission, one-third of patients with acute *P. falciparum* infection are co-infected with *P. vivax*, and 8% of patients with acute vivax malaria have simultaneous *P. falciparum* infection. Mixed infections are underestimated by routine microscopy. Cryptic *P. falciparum* infections can be revealed in approximately 75% of cases by the RDTs based on the histidine-rich protein 2 (HRP2) antigen, but such antigen tests are much less useful (because of their lower sensitivity) in detecting cryptic vivax malaria. ACTs are effective against all malaria species and are the treatment of choice. Radical treatment with primaquine should be given to patients with confirmed *P. vivax* and *P. ovale* infections except in high transmission settings where the risk of re-infection is high.

11. COMPLEX EMERGENCIES AND EPIDEMICS

When large numbers of people are displaced within malaria endemic areas there is an increased risk of a malaria epidemic, especially when people living in an area with little or no malaria transmission move to an endemic area (e.g. displacement from highland to lowland areas). The lack of protective immunity, concentration of population, breakdown in public health activities and difficulties in accessing insecticides, insecticide-treated nets and effective treatment, all conspire to fuel epidemic malaria, in which morbidity and mortality are often high. Such circumstances are also ideal for the development of resistance to antimalarials. For these reasons, particular efforts must be made to deliver effective antimalarial treatment to the population at risk.

11.1 Diagnosis

In epidemic and complex emergency situations, facilities for laboratory diagnosis may be either unavailable or so overwhelmed with the case-load that parasite-based diagnosis is impossible. In such circumstances, it is impractical and unnecessary to demonstrate parasites before treatment in all cases of fever. Once an epidemic of malaria has been confirmed, and if case numbers are high, treatment based solely on the clinical history is appropriate in most cases, using a full treatment course. However, parasite-based diagnosis is essential to:
- diagnose the cause of an epidemic of febrile illness,
- monitor and confirm the end of an epidemic,
- follow progress in infants, pregnant women, and those with severe malaria.

As the epidemic wanes, the proportion of fever cases investigated parasitologically can be increased. It is important to monitor the clinical response to treatment wherever possible, bearing in mind that other infections may also be present. In mixed falciparum/vivax epidemics, parasitaemia should be monitored in order to determine a species-specific treatment.

11.2 Use of rapid diagnostic tests in epidemic situations

RDTs offer the advantage of simplicity and speed in epidemic situations, but heat stability may be a problem and false-negative results may be seen. A negative result should not automatically preclude treatment, especially in severe clinical disease. Current experience with RDTs indicates that they are useful for confirming the cause and end-point of malaria epidemics, but they should not be relied on as the sole basis for treatment. They should also be backed up with adequate quality assurance, including temperature stability testing.

11.3   Management of uncomplicated malaria in epidemics

Malaria epidemics are emergencies in which populations at risk in epidemic-prone areas are mainly non-immune or only partially immune. The principles of treatment are the same as elsewhere (see section 7); the antimalarial to be used in epidemics (and complex emergencies) must be highly efficacious (≥95% cure), safe and well tolerated so that adherence to treatment is high. Complete courses of treatment should always be given in all circumstances.

The rapid and reliable antimalarial effects of ACTs and their gametocytocidal properties, which reduce transmission, make them ideal for treatment in a malaria epidemic. An active search should be made for febrile patients to ensure that, as many cases as possible are treated, rather than relying on patients to come to a clinic.

Summary of recommendations on treatment of uncomplicated malaria in epidemic situations

RECOMMENDATIONS	LEVEL OF EVIDENCE
ACTs are recommended for antimalarial treatment in epidemics in all areas with the exception of countries in Central America and the Island of Hispaniola, where chloroquine and sulfadoxine-pyrimethamine still have a very high efficacy against falciparum malaria. Chloroquine 25 mg base/kg bw divided over 3 days, combined with primaquine 0.25 mg base/kg bw, taken with food once a day for 14 days is the treatment of choice for chloroquine-sensitive *P. vivax* infections. In Oceania and South-East Asia the dose of primaquine should be 0.5 mg/kg bw.	O, E
In situations where ACTs are not immediately available, the most effective alternative should be used until ACTs become available.	O, E

11.4   Areas prone to mixed falciparum/vivax malaria epidemics

Resistance of *P. vivax* to chloroquine has been reported from South-East Asia and Oceania but is probably limited in distribution. There is insufficient knowledge at present to allow specific recommendations to be made for treatment of *P. vivax* epidemics in areas of suspected resistance. ACTs (except artesunate + sulfadoxine-pyrimethamine) should be used for treatment as they are highly effective against all malaria species. In areas with pure vivax epidemics, and where drug resistance has not been reported, chloroquine is the most appropriate drug once the cause of the epidemic has been established.

11.5   Use of gametocytocidal drugs to reduce transmission

ACTs reduce gametocyte carriage markedly, and therefore reduce transmission. This is very valuable in epidemic control. In the only randomized comparison reported, ACTs had a greater effect than primaquine on gametocyte carriage. In circumstances where an ACT is not used, a single oral dose of primaquine of 0.75 mg base/kg bw (45 mg base maximal for adults) combined with a fully effective blood schizonticide could be used to reduce transmission provided that it is possible to achieve high coverage (> 85%) of the population infected with malaria. This strategy has been widely used in South-East Asia and South America, although its impact has not been well documented. The single primaquine dose was well tolerated and prior testing for G6PD deficiency was not required. There is no experience with its use in Africa, where there is the highest prevalence of G6PD deficiency in the world. Primaquine should not be given in pregnancy. Whether there is any additional benefit in combining primaquine with an ACT is unknown. There is insufficient evidence to recommend this.

11.6   Anti-relapse therapy in vivax malaria epidemics

Anti-relapse therapy for vivax malaria is impractical in most epidemic situations because of the duration of treatment and poor compliance. If adequate records are kept, it can be given in the post-epidemic period to patients who have been treated with blood schizonticides. Primaquine 0.25–0.5 mg base/kg bw daily doses should be given for 14 days, as there is no evidence that shorter courses are effective. Compliance with radical (anti-relapse) treatment is often poor and the drug should ideally be given under supervision, which is very difficult in epidemic situations. Appropriate health education should be provided to assist malaria control and encourage adherence.

11.7   Mass treatment

Mass treatment (mass drug administration) of all or a large section of the population whether symptoms are present or not) has been carried out in the past, usually in conjunction with insecticide residual spraying, as a way of controlling epidemics. Analysis of 19 mass drug administration projects during the period 1932–1999 did not draw definitive conclusions because study designs were so variable.[20] Many projects were unsuccessful, although a

---

[20] von Seidlein L, Greenwood BM. Mass administration of antimalarial drugs. *Trends in Parasitology*, 2003, 19:790–796.

reduction in parasite prevalence and some transient reduction in mortality and morbidity occurred in some cases. Reduced transmission was seen only in one study, in Vanuatu, where the population concerned was relatively small, well defined and controlled.

There is no convincing evidence for the benefits of mass treatment. Mass treatment of symptomatic febrile patients is considered appropriate in epidemic and complex emergency situations. Whenever this strategy is adopted, a full treatment course should be given.

LIST OF ANNEXES

ANNEX 1

THE GUIDELINES DEVELOPMENT PROCESS

A1.1 Treatment recommendations

The *WHO Guidelines for the Treatment of Malaria* were developed in accordance with the guidance established by WHO for the formulation of such guidelines.[21]

The development process was undertaken at a technical consultation on malaria treatment guidelines and by the Technical Guidelines Development Group, chaired by Professor Nick White (participants are listed below). Conflict of interest statements were received from all participants, and no conflict of interest was declared by any of the participants. The first technical consultation was convened in April 2004, at which the target audience for the guidelines was defined and the scope of the guidelines and key questions to be addressed were determined.

Following the first meeting, contracts for systematic search and reviews of relevant evidence were awarded to research groups from two institutions: the Liverpool School of Tropical Medicine, Liverpool, England and Mahidol University, Bangkok, Thailand. The search strategies employed included a search of the following databases:

- the Cochrane Infectious Diseases Group trials register (up to June 2004),*
- the Cochrane Central Register of Controlled Trials (CENTRAL) published in The Cochrane Library (Issue 2, 2004),*
- MEDLINE (1966 to June 2004),
- EMBASE (1980 to June 2004),
- LILACS (1982 to June 2004).

The evidence for RCTs was assembled in collaboration with Clinical Evidence, a product of BMJ Knowledge.

The following search terms were used:

- malaria (free text),
- malaria (controlled vocabulary, MESH or EMTREE).

The terms were used in combination with the search strategy for retrieving randomized and controlled clinical trials developed by The Cochrane Collaboration. Key words relative to currently available antimalarial drugs were used for

---

[21] *Guidelines for guidelines.* Geneva, World Health Organization, 2003 (document EIP/GPE/EQC/2003.1).

each section of the review. Where indicated, specific authors and research groups were contacted for more information on published work and work in progress.

In formulating recommendations, evidence was graded in order of priority as follows:

- formal systematic reviews, such as Cochrane reviews, including more than one randomized control trial,
- comparative trials without formal systematic review,
- observational studies (e.g. surveillance, pharmacological data),
- expert opinion/consensus.

The Technical Guidelines Development Group held its first meeting in August 2004 and produced a preliminary draft that was presented and revised at the second technical consultation in October 2004. The revised draft of the guidelines was sent out for external peer review in November 2004. At a subsequent meeting of the Technical Guidelines Development Group in January 2005, the document was revised further in the light of comments received. The Guidelines development process and publication was fully funded by WHO. It is planned that the evidence will be reviewed on an annual basis, and that the guidelines will be updated periodically. Similarly a mechanism for periodic monitoring and evaluating the use of the treatment guidelines in countries would be established.

A1.2 Members of the Technical Guidelines Development Group

Temporary advisers

Dr D. Baza, National Malaria Control Programme Manager, Ministry of Health, Burundi

Dr D. Bethell*, Faculty of Tropical Medicine, Mahidol University, Bangkok, Thailand

Professor A. Bjorkman, Division of Infectious Diseases, Karolinska University Hospital, Stockholm, Sweden

Professor M. Boulos, Hospital das Clinicas da Faculdade de Medicina da Universidade de São Paulo, São Paulo, Brazil

Professor M. A. Faiz, Department of Medicine, Dhaka Medical College, Bangladesh

Professor P. Garner*, Liverpool School of Tropical Medicine,
Liverpool, England

Professor O. Gaye, Service de Parasitologie, Faculté de Médecine,
Université Cheikh Anta Diop, Dakar-Fann, Senegal

Dr T. Ghebremeskel, National Malaria Programme Manager, Ministry
of Health, Asmara, Eritrea

Dr S. Hill*, Discipline of Clinical Pharmacology, Faculty of Medicine &
Health Sciences, University of Newcastle, Newcastle Mater Hospital,
Newcastle, Australia

Dr K. Jones*, Clinical Research Fellow, Liverpool School of Tropical
Medicine, Liverpool, England

Dr S. Lutalo, Consultant Physician, Harare Central Hospital,
Harare, Zimbabwe

Dr A. McCarthy, Director, Tropical Medicine and International Division of
Infectious Diseases, Ottawa Hospital General Campus, Ottawa, Canada

Dr O. Mokuolu*, Consultant Paediatrician, University of Ilorin Teaching
Hospital, Ilorin, Nigeria

Dr S. Nyirenda, Consultant Physician, Department of Medicine,
University Teaching Hospital, Lusaka, Zambia

Dr E. Tjitra*, Senior Researcher, National Institute of Health
& Development, Ministry of Health, Jakarta, Indonesia

Dr L.S. Vestergaard, Laboratory of Parasitic Diseases, Statens Serum
Institut, and Department of International Health, University of
Copenhagen, Copenhagen, Denmark

Professor N. White* (*Chairman*) Faculty of Tropical Medicine,
Mahidol University, Bangkok, Thailand

WHO Secretariat

Dr D. Bell, Malaria and Parasitic Diseases, WHO Regional Office for
the Western Pacific, Manila, Philippines

Dr A. Bosman, Roll Back Malaria Department, World Health Organization,
Geneva, Switzerland

Dr C. Delacollette, Roll Back Malaria Department, World Health
Organization, Geneva, Switzerland

Dr M. Gomes, UNDP/UNICEF/World Bank/WHO Special Programme for
Research and Training in Tropical Diseases, World Health Organization,
Geneva, Switzerland

Dr R. Gray, Essential Drugs and Medicine, World Health Organization, Geneva, Switzerland

Dr K.N. Mendis*, Roll Back Malaria Department, World Health Organization, Geneva, Switzerland

Dr F. Nafo-Traoré, Roll Back Malaria Department, World Health Organization, Geneva, Switzerland

Dr B.L. Nahlen, Roll Back Malaria Department, World Health Organization, Geneva, Switzerland

Dr P.E. Olumese* (*Secretary*), Roll Back Malaria Department, World Health Organization, Geneva, Switzerland

Dr C. Ondari*, Essential Drugs and Medicine, World Health Organization, Geneva, Switzerland

Dr R. Ridley*, UNDP/UNICEF/World Bank/WHO Special Programme for Research and Training in Tropical Diseases, World Health Organization, Geneva, Switzerland

Dr A.E.C. Rietveld*, Roll Back Malaria Department, World Health Organization, Geneva, Switzerland

Dr P. Ringwald, Roll Back Malaria Department, World Health Organization, Geneva, Switzerland

Dr I. Sanou, Malaria, WHO Regional Office for Africa, Harare, Zimbabwe.

Dr A. Schapira, Roll Back Malaria Department, World Health Organization, Geneva, Switzerland

Dr T. Sukwa*, Malaria, WHO Regional Office for Africa, Harare, Zimbabwe

Dr T. Tantorres, Evidence and Information for Policy, World Health Organization, Geneva, Switzerland

Dr W. Taylor, UNDP/UNICEF/World Bank/WHO Special Programme for Research and Training in Tropical Diseases, World Health Organization, Geneva, Switzerland

Dr Y. Touré, UNDP/UNICEF/World Bank/WHO Special Programme for Research and Training in Tropical Diseases, World Health Organization, Geneva, Switzerland

Dr W.M. Were, Roll Back Malaria Department, World Health Organization, Geneva, Switzerland

---

* Members of the Guidelines drafting committee.

Annex 2. Adaptation of *WHO malaria treatment guidelines* for use in countries

ANNEX 2

ADAPTATION OF *WHO MALARIA TREATMENT GUIDELINES* FOR USE IN COUNTRIES

A2.1   Background

WHO has recently convened technical consultations aimed at developing guidelines for the treatment of malaria.[22]

The guidelines are generic in nature and should therefore be adapted by regions and countries alike to take account of local conditions, especially when formulating implementation and scale-up strategies.

A number of malaria endemic countries have not yet elaborated national malaria treatment guidelines, although treatment protocols may be available at the health-care provider level. Furthermore, existing national guidelines need to be updated as many countries, especially in sub-Saharan Africa, are adopting and starting to implement policies specifying the use of artemisinin combination therapies (ACTs).

This annex provides orientation and guidance on the process countries should follow in adapting the content of the generic malaria treatment guidelines provided in the main document.

A2.2   The development process

The ministry of health should take the lead in the process of developing national malaria treatment guidelines.[23]

The proposed steps include the following.

- *A national workshop on the malaria treatment guidelines* is the first step at country level. This workshop will review any current national malaria treatment guidelines, identify specific issues that need to be addressed and provide major policy recommendations.
- *Drafting/updating the national malaria treatment guidelines*. Following the national workshop, the national malaria case management committee (or its equivalent) should spearhead the development of new national malaria treatment guidelines in accordance with the standard outline set out below.

---

[22] The guidelines development process is described in Annex 1.

[23] The preparation of the treatment guidelines is only one component of implementation of antimalarial treatment policy.

- *A consensus workshop on the national malaria treatment guidelines* should then be arranged to present, discuss and adopt the draft national malaria treatment guidelines.
- *Finalization and dissemination.* The national malaria treatment guidelines are finalized, officially endorsed and disseminated.

A2.3 The content

It is recommended that national malaria treatment guidelines are presented in a similar way as WHO Guidelines on the Treatment of Malaria. The following outline is suggested:

1. General introduction
   - Epidemiological situation and parasite distribution
   - National drug resistance pattern

2. Diagnosis of malaria
   - Clinical diagnosis
   - Role of parasitological diagnosis

3. Treatment of *P. falciparum* malaria or the most prevalent species in the country
   - Uncomplicated malaria
     - definition
     - treatment objectives
     - treatment recommendations
     - treatment in specific populations and situations
   - Severe malaria
     - definition
     - treatment objectives
     - treatment recommendations
     - pre-referral treatment options
     - management in epidemic situations

4. Treatment of malaria caused by other species

5. Disease management at the different levels of the health care delivery system

6. Annexes – Relevant annexes should be attached to provide more detailed information on, for example, dosages of drugs, specific data on therapeutic efficacy of antimalarial medicines in the country, other available evidence for treatment recommendation, etc.

ANNEX 3

PHARMACOLOGY OF ANTIMALARIAL DRUGS

A3.1   Chloroquine

Molecular weight: 436.0

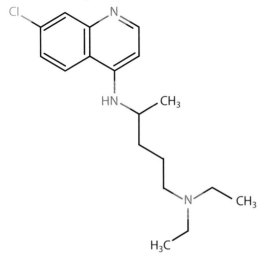

Chloroquine is a 4-aminoquinoline that has been used extensively for the treatment and prevention of malaria. Widespread resistance has now rendered it virtually useless against *P. falciparum* infections in most parts of the world, although it still maintains considerable efficacy for the treatment of *P. vivax*, *P. ovale* and *P. malariae* infections. As with other 4-aminoquinolines, it does not produce radical cure.

Chloroquine interferes with parasite haem detoxification *(1, 2)*. Resistance is related to genetic changes in transporters (PfCRT, PfMDR), which reduce the concentrations of chloroquine at its site of action, the parasite food vacuole.

Formulations
- Tablets containing 100 mg or 150 mg of chloroquine base as hydrochloride, phosphate or sulfate.

Pharmacokinetics
Chloroquine is rapidly and almost completely absorbed from the gastrointestinal tract when taken orally, although peak plasma concentrations can vary considerably. Absorption is also very rapid following intramuscular and subcutaneous

administration *(3–5)*. Chloroquine is extensively distributed into body tissues, including the placenta and breast milk, and has an enormous total apparent volume of distribution. The relatively small volume of distribution of the central compartment means that transiently cardiotoxic levels may occur following intravenous administration unless the rate of parenteral delivery is strictly controlled. Some 60% of chloroquine is bound to plasma proteins, and the drug is eliminated slowly from the body via the kidneys, with an estimated terminal elimination half-life of 1–2 months. Chloroquine is metabolized in the liver, mainly to monodesethylchloroquine, which has similar activity against *P. falciparum*.

Toxicity

Chloroquine has a low safety margin and is very dangerous in overdosage. Larger doses of chloroquine are used for the treatment of rheumatoid arthritis than for malaria, so adverse effects are seen more frequently in patients with arthritis. The drug is generally well tolerated. The principle limiting adverse effects in practice are the unpleasant taste, which may upset children, and pruritus, which may be severe in dark-skinned patients *(6)*. Other less common side effects include headache, various skin eruptions and gastrointestinal disturbances, such as nausea, vomiting and diarrhoea. More rarely central nervous system toxicity including, convulsions and mental changes may occur. Chronic use (>5 years continuous use as prophylaxis) may lead to eye disorders, including keratopathy and retinopathy. Other uncommon effects include myopathy, reduced hearing, photosensitivity and loss of hair. Blood disorders, such as aplastic anaemia, are extremely uncommon *(7)*.

Acute overdosage is extremely dangerous and death can occur within a few hours. The patient may progress from feeling dizzy and drowsy with headache and gastrointestinal upset, to developing sudden visual disturbance, convulsions, hypokalaemia, hypotension and cardiac arrhythmias. There is no specific treatment, although diazepam and epinephrine (adrenaline) administered together are beneficial *(8, 9)*.

Drug interactions

Major interactions are very unusual. There is a theoretical increased risk of arrhythmias when chloroquine is given with halofantrine or other drugs that prolong the electrocardiograph QT interval; a possible increased risk of convulsions with mefloquine; reduced absorption with antacids; reduced metabolism and clearance with cimetidine; an increased risk of acute dystonic reactions with metronidazole; reduced bioavailability of ampicillin and praziquantel; reduced therapeutic effect of thyroxine; a possible antagonistic effect on the antiepileptic effects of carbamazepine and sodium valproate; and increased plasma concentrations of cyclosporine.

A3.2 Amodiaquine

Molecular weight: 355.9

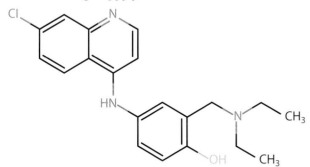

Amodiaquine is a Mannich base 4-aminoquinoline with a mode of action similar to that of chloroquine. It is effective against some chloroquine-resistant strains of *P. falciparum*, although there is cross-resistance.

Formulations

• Tablets containing 200 mg of amodiaquine base as hydrochloride or 153.1 mg of base as chlorohydrate.

Pharmacokinetics

Amodiaquine hydrochloride is readily absorbed from the gastrointestinal tract. It is rapidly converted in the liver to the active metabolite desethylamodiaquine, which contributes nearly all of the antimalarial effect *(10)*. There are insufficient data on the terminal plasma elimination half-life of desethylamodiaquine. Both amodiaquine and desethylamodiaquine have been detected in the urine several months after administration.

Toxicity

The adverse effects of amodiaquine are similar to those of chloroquine. Amodiaquine is associated with less pruritus and is more palatable than chloroquine, but is associated with a much higher risk of agranulocytosis and, to a lesser degree, of hepatitis when used for prophylaxis *(11)*. The risk of a serious adverse reaction with prophylactic use (which is no longer recommended) appears to be between 1 in 1000 and 1 in 5000. It is not clear whether the risks are lower when amodiaquine is used to treat malaria. Following overdose cardiotoxicity appears to be less frequent than with chloroquine. Large doses of amodiaquine have been reported to cause syncope, spasticity, convulsions and involuntary movements.

Drug interactions

There are insufficient data.

A3.3   Sulfadoxine

Molecular weight: 310.3

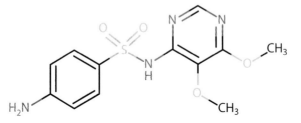

Sulfadoxine is a slowly eliminated sulfonamide. It is very slightly soluble in water. Sulfonamides are structural analogues and competitive antagonists of *p*-aminobenzoic acid. They are competitive inhibitors of dihydropteroate synthase, the bacterial enzyme responsible for the incorporation of *p*-aminobenzoic acid in the synthesis of folic acid.

Formulations

Sulfadoxine is used in a fixed-dose combination of 20 parts sulfadoxine with 1 part pyrimethamine and may be administered orally or by the intramuscular route:

- Tablets containing 500 mg of sulfadoxine and 25 mg of pyrimethamine.
- Ampoules containing 500 mg of sulfadoxine and 25 mg of pyrimethamine in 2.5 ml of injectable solution for intramuscular use.

Pharmacokinetics

Sulfadoxine is readily absorbed from the gastrointestinal tract. Peak blood concentrations occur about 4 h after an oral dose. The terminal elimination half-life is 4–9 days. Around 90–95% is bound to plasma proteins. It is widely distributed to body tissues and fluids, passes into the fetal circulation and is detectable in breast milk. The drug is excreted in urine, primarily unchanged.

Toxicity

Sulfadoxine shares the adverse effect profile of other sulfonamides, although allergic reactions can be severe because of its slow elimination. Nausea, vomiting, anorexia and diarrhoea may occur. Crystalluria causing lumbar pain, haematuria and oliguria is rare compared with more rapidly eliminated sulphonamides. Hypersensitivity reactions may effect different organ system. Cutaneous manifestations can be severe and include pruritus, photosensitivity reactions, exfoliative dermatitis, erythema nodosum, toxic epidermal necrolysis and Stevens-Johnson syndrome (12). Treatment with sulfadoxine should be stopped in any patient developing a rash because of the risk of severe allergic reactions (13). Hypersensitivity to sulfadoxine may also cause interstitial nephritis, lumbar pain, haematuria and oliguria. This is due to crystal formation in the urine (crystalluria) and may be avoided by keeping the patient well hydrated to maintain a high urine output. Alkalinization of the urine will also make the crystals more soluble. Blood disorders that have been reported include agranulocytosis, aplastic anaemia, thrombocytopenia, leukopenia and hypoprothrombinaemia. Acute haemolytic anaemia is a rare complication, which may be antibody mediated or associated with glucose-6-phosphate dehydrogenase (G6PD) deficiency. Other adverse effects, which may be mani-festations of a generalized hypersensitivity reaction include fever, interstitial nephritis, a syndrome resembling serum sickness, hepatitis, myocarditis, pul-monary eosinophilia, fibrosing alveolitis, peripheral neuropathy and systemic vasculitis, including polyarteritis nodosa. Anaphylaxis has been reported only rarely. Other adverse reactions that have been reported include hypo-glycaemia, jaundice in neonates, aseptic meningitis, drowsiness, fatigue, headache, ataxia, dizziness, drowsiness, convulsions, neuropathies, psychosis and pseudomembranous colitis.

A3.4 Pyrimethamine

Molecular weight: 248.7

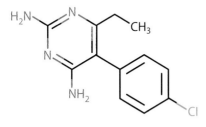

Pyrimethamine is a diaminopyrimidine used in combination with a sulfonamide, usually sulfadoxine or dapsone. It exerts its antimalarial activity by inhibiting plasmodial dihydrofolate reductase thus indirectly blocking the synthesis of nucleic acids in the malaria parasite. It is a slow-acting blood schizontocide and is also possibly active against pre-erythrocytic forms of the malaria parasite and inhibits sporozoite development in the mosquito vector. It is effective against all four human malarias, although resistance has emerged rapidly. Pyrimethamine is also used in the treatment of toxoplasmosis, and isosporiasis and as prophylaxis against *Pneumocystis carinii* pneumonia. Pyrimethamine is no longer used alone as an antimalarial, only in synergistic combination with slowly eliminated sulfonamides for treatment (sulfadoxine, sulfalene) or with dapsone for prophylaxis.

Formulations

Pyrimethamine is currently used mainly in a fixed-dose combination with slowly eliminated sulfonamides, either of 20 parts sulfadoxine with 1 part pyrimethamine for which there are oral and parenteral formulations:

- Tablets containing 500 mg of sulfadoxine and 25 mg of pyrimethamine.
- Ampoules containing 500 mg of sulfadoxine and 25 mg of pyrimethamine in 2.5 ml of injectable solution for intramuscular use.

Pharmacokinetics

Pyrimethamine is almost completely absorbed from the gastrointestinal tract and peak plasma concentrations occur 2–6 h after an oral dose. It is mainly concentrated in the kidneys, lungs, liver and spleen, and about 80–90% is bound to plasma proteins. It is metabolized in the liver and slowly excreted via the kidneys. The plasma half-life is around 4 days. Pyrimethamine crosses the blood-brain barrier and the placenta and is detectable in breast milk. Absorption of the intramuscular preparation is incomplete and insufficiently reliable for this formulation to be recommended *(14)*.

Toxicity

Pyrimethamine is generally very well tolerated. Administration for prolonged periods may cause depression of haematopoiesis due to interference with folic acid metabolism. Skin rashes and hypersensitivity reactions also occur. Larger doses may cause gastrointestinal symptoms such as atrophic glossitis, abdominal pain and vomiting, haematological effects including megaloblastic anaemia, leukopenia, thrombocytopenia and pancytopenia, and central nervous system effects such as headache and dizziness.

Acute overdosage of pyrimethamine can cause gastrointestinal effects and stimulation of the central nervous system with vomiting, excitability and convulsions. Tachycardia, respiratory depression, circulatory collapse and death may follow. Treatment of overdosage is supportive.

Drug interactions

Administration of pyrimethamine with other folate antagonists such as cotri-moxazole, trimethoprim, methotrexate or with phenytoin may exacerbate bone marrow depression. Given with some benzodiazepines, there is a risk of hepatotoxicity.

A3.5 Mefloquine

Molecular weight: 378.3

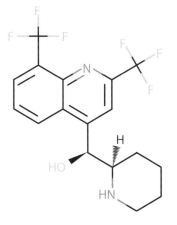

Mefloquine is a 4-methanolquinoline and is related to quinine. It is soluble in alcohol but only very slightly soluble in water. It should be protected from light. The drug is effective against all forms of malaria.

Formulations

Mefloquine is administered by mouth as the hydrochloride salt (250 mg base equivalent to 274 mg hydrochloride salt):

- Tablets containing either 250 mg salt (United States of America) or 250 mg base (elsewhere).

Pharmacokinetics

Mefloquine is reasonably well absorbed from the gastrointestinal tract but there is marked interindividual variation in the time required to achieve peak plasma concentrations. Splitting the 25 mg/kg dose into two parts given at an interval of 6–24 h augments absorption and improves tolerability *(15)*. Mefloquine undergoes enterohepatic recycling. It is approximately 98% bound to plasma proteins and is widely distributed throughout the body. The pharmacokinetics of mefloquine may be altered by malaria infection with reduced absorption and accelerated clearance *(16, 17)*. When administered with artesunate, blood concentrations are increased, probably as an indirect effect of increased absorption resulting from more rapid resolution of symptoms *(15)*. Mefloquine is excreted in small amounts in breast milk. It has a long elimination half-life of around 21 days, which is shortened in malaria to about 14 days, possibly because of interrupted enterohepatic cycling *(18–20)*. Mefloquine is metabolized in the liver and excreted mainly in the bile and faeces. Its pharmacokinetics show enantioselectivity after administration of the racemic mixture, with higher peak plasma concentrations and area under the curve values, and lower volume of distribution and total clearance of the SR enantiomer than its RS antipode *(21–23)*.

Toxicity

Minor adverse effects are common following mefloquine treatment, most frequently nausea, vomiting, abdominal pain, anorexia, diarrhoea, headache, dizziness, loss of balance, dysphoria, somnolence and sleep disorders, notably insomnia and abnormal dreams. Neuropsychiatric disturbances (seizures, encephalopathy, psychosis) occur in approximately 1 in 10 000 travellers receiving mefloquine prophylaxis, 1 in 1000 patients treated in Asia, 1 in 200 patients treated in Africa, and 1 in 20 patients following severe malaria *(24–27)*. Other side effects reported rarely include skin rashes, pruritus and urticaria, hair loss, muscle weakness, liver function disturbances and very rarely thrombocytopenia and leukopenia. Cardiovascular effects have included postural hypotension, bradycardia and, rarely, hypertension, tachycardia or palpitations and minor changes in the electrocardiogram. Fatalities have not been reported following overdosage, although cardiac, hepatic and neurological symptoms may be seen. Mefloquine should not be given with halofantrine because it exacerbates QT prolongation. There is no evidence of an adverse interaction with quinine *(28)*.

Drug interactions

There is a possible increase in the risk of arrhythmias if mefloquine is given together with beta blockers, calcium channel blockers, amiodarone, pimozide, digoxin or antidepressants; there is also a possible increase in the risk of convulsions with chloroquine and quinine. Mefloquine concentrations are increased when given with ampicillin, tetracycline and metoclopramide. Caution should be observed with alcohol.

A3.6   Artemisinin and its derivatives

A3.6.1   Artemisinin

Molecular weight: 282.3

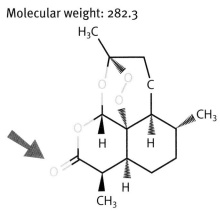

Artemisinin, also known as qinghaosu, is a sesquiterpene lactone extracted from the leaves of *Artemisia annua* (sweet wormwood). It has been used in China for the treatment of fever for over a thousand years. It is a potent and rapidly acting blood schizontocide and is active against all *Plasmodium* species. It has an unusually broad activity against asexual parasites, killing all stages from young rings to schizonts. In *P. falciparum* malaria, artemisinin also kills the gametocytes – including the stage 4 gametocytes, which are otherwise sensitive only to primaquine. Artemisinin and its derivatives inhibit an essential calcium adenosine triphosphatase, PfATPase 6 *(29)*. Artemisinin has now largely given way to the more potent dihydroartemisinin and its derivatives, artemether, artemotil and artesunate. The three latter derivatives are converted back *in vivo* to dihydroartemisinin. These drugs should be given as combination therapy to protect them from resistance.

Formulations

A wide variety of formulations for oral, parenteral and rectal use are available. These include:

- Tablets and capsules containing 250 mg of artemisinin.
- Suppositories containing 100 mg, 200 mg, 300 mg, 400 mg or 500 mg of artemisinin.

Pharmacokinetics

Peak plasma concentrations occur around 3 h and 11 h following oral and rectal administration respectively *(30)*. Artemisinin is converted to inactive metabolites via the cytochrome P450 enzyme CYP2B6 and other enzymes.

Artemisinin is a potent inducer of its own metabolism. The elimination half-life is approximately 1 h *(31)*.

Toxicity

Artemisinin and its derivatives are safe and remarkably well tolerated *(32, 33)*. There have been reports of mild gastrointestinal disturbances, dizziness, tinnitus, reticulocytopenia, neutropenia, elevated liver enzyme values, and electrocardiographic abnormalities, including bradycardia and prolongation of the QT interval, although most studies have not found any electrocardiographic abnormalities. The only potentially serious adverse effect reported with this class of drugs is type 1 hypersensitivity reactions in approximately 1 in 3000 patients *(34)*. Neurotoxicity has been reported in animal studies, particularly with very high doses of intramuscular artemotil and artemether, but has not been substantiated in humans *(35–37)*. Similarly, evidence of death of embryos and morphological abnormalities in early pregnancy have been demonstrated in animal studies (37a). Artemisinin has not been evaluated in the first trimester of pregnancy so should be avoided in first trimester patients with uncomplicated malaria until more information is available.

Drug interactions

None known.

A3.6.2 Artemether

Molecular weight: 298.4

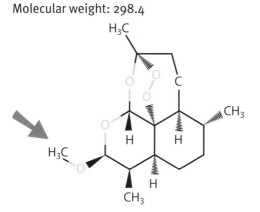

Artemether is the methyl ether of dihydroartemisinin. It is more lipid soluble than artemisinin or artesunate. It can be given as an oil-based intramuscular injection or orally. It is also coformulated with lumefantrine (previously referred to as benflumetol) for combination therapy.

Formulations

- Capsules containing 40 mg of artemether.
- Tablets containing 50 mg of artemether.
- Ampoules of injectable solution for intramuscular injection containing 80 mg of artemether in 1 ml for adults or 40 mg of artemether in 1 ml for paediatric use.

In a coformulation with lumefantrine:

- Tablets containing 20 mg of artemether and 120 mg of lumefantrine.

Pharmacokinetics

Peak plasma concentrations occur around 2–3 h after oral administration *(38)*. Following intramuscular injection, absorption is very variable, especially in children with poor peripheral perfusion: peak plasma concentrations generally occur after around 6 h but absorption is slow and erratic and times to peak can be 18 h or longer in some cases *(39–41)*. Artemether is metabolized to dihydroartemisinin, the active metabolite. After intramuscular administration, artemether predominates, whereas after oral administration dihydroartemisinin predominates. Biotransformation is mediated via the cytochrome P450 enzyme CYP3A4. Autoinduction of metabolism is less than with artemisinin. Artemether is 95% bound to plasma proteins. The elimination half-life is approximately 1 h, but following intramuscular administration the elimination phase is prolonged because of continued absorption. No dose modifications are necessary in renal or hepatic impairment.

Toxicity

In all species of animals tested, intramuscular artemether and artemotil cause an unusual selective pattern of neuronal damage to certain brain stem nuclei. Neurotoxicity in experimental animals is related to the sustained blood concentrations that follow intramuscular administration *(42)*, since it is much less frequent when the same doses are given orally, or with similar doses of water-soluble drugs such as artesunate. Clinical, neurophysiological and pathological studies in humans have not shown similar findings with therapeutic use of these compounds *(40)*. Toxicity is otherwise similar to that of artemisinin.

Drug interactions

None known.

A3.6.3 Artesunate
Molecular weight: 384.4

Artesunate is the sodium salt of the hemisuccinate ester of artemisinin. It is soluble in water but has poor stability in aqueous solutions at neutral or acid pH. In the injectable form, artesunic acid is drawn up in sodium bicarbonate to form sodium artesunate immediately before injection. Artesunate can be given orally, rectally or by the intramuscular or intravenous routes. There are no coformulations currently available.

Formulations
- Tablets containing 50 mg or 200 mg of sodium artesunate.
- Ampoules: intramuscular or intravenous injection containing 60 mg of anhydrous artesunic acid with a separate ampoule of 5% sodium bicarbonate solution.
- Rectal capsules containing 100 mg or 400 mg of sodium artesunate.

Pharmacokinetics
Artesunate is rapidly absorbed, with peak plasma levels occurring 1.5 h and 2 h and 0.5 h after oral, rectal and intramuscular administration, respectively *(43–47)*. It is almost entirely converted to dihydroartemisinin, the active metabolite *(30)*. Elimination of artesunate is very rapid, and antimalarial activity is determined by dihydroartemisinin elimination (half-life approximately 45 min) *(40)*. The extent of protein binding is unknown. No dose modifications are necessary in renal or hepatic impairment.

Toxicity
As for artemisinin.

Drug interactions
None known.

A3.6.4 Dihydroartemisinin

Molecular weight: 284.4

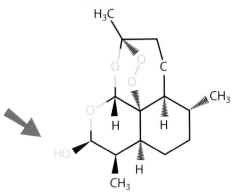

Dihydroartemisinin is the main active metabolite of the artemisinin derivatives, but can also be given orally and rectally as a drug in its own right. It is relatively insoluble in water, and requires formulation with suitable excipients to ensure adequate absorption. It achieves cure rates similar to those of oral artesunate. A fixed-dose formulation with piperaquine is currently undergoing evaluation as a promising new artemisinin-based combination therapy (ACT).

Formulations

- Tablets containing 20 mg, 60 mg or 80 mg of dihydroartemisinin.
- Suppositories containing 80 mg of dihydroartemisinin.

Pharmacokinetics

Dihydroartemisinin is rapidly absorbed following oral administration, reaching peak levels after around 2.5 h. Absorption via the rectal route is somewhat slower, with peak levels occurring around 4 h after administration. Plasma protein binding is around 55%. Elimination half-life is approximately 45 min via intestinal and hepatic glucuronidation (48).

Toxicity

As for artemisinin.

Drug interactions

None known.

A3.6.5 Artemotil

Molecular weight: 312.4

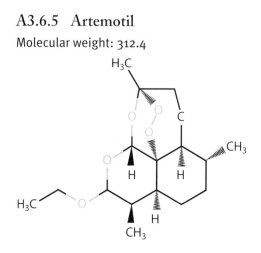

Artemotil, previously known as arteether, is the ethyl ether of artemisinin, and is closely related to the more widely used artemether. It is oil-based so water insoluble. It is given by intramuscular injection only.

Formulations

• Ampoules containing 150 mg of artemotil in 2 ml of injectable solution.

Pharmacokinetics

There is less published information on artemotil than for artemether. Absorption is slower and more erratic, with some patients having undetectable plasma artemotil until more than 24 h after administration.

Toxicity

As for artemisinin.

Drug interactions

None known.

A3.7 Lumefantrine (benflumetol)

Molecular weight: 528.9

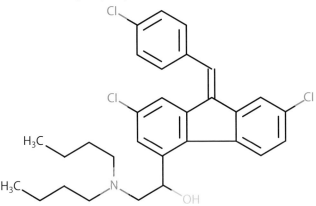

Lumefantrine belongs to the aryl aminoalcohol group of antimalarials, which also includes quinine, mefloquine and halofantrine. It has a similar mechanism of action. Lumefantrine is a racemic fluorine derivative developed in China. It is only available in an oral preparation coformulated with artemether. This ACT is highly effective against multidrug-resistant *P. falciparum*.

Formulations

Available only in an oral preparation coformulated with artemether:

• Tablets containing 20 mg of artemether and 120 mg of lumefantrine.

Pharmacokinetics

Oral bioavailability is variable and is highly dependant on administration with fatty foods *(38, 49)*. Absorption increases by 108% after a meal and is lower in patients with acute malaria than in convalescing patients. Peak plasma levels occur approximately 10 h after administration. The terminal elimination half-life is around 3 days.

Toxicity

Despite similarities with the structure and pharmacokinetic properties of halofantrine, lumefantrine does not significantly prolong the electrocardio-graphic QT interval, and has no other significant toxicity *(50)*. In fact the drug seems to be remarkably well tolerated. Reported side effects are generally mild – nausea, abdominal discomfort, headache and dizziness – and cannot be distinguished from symptoms of acute malaria.

Drug interactions

The manufacturer of artemether-lumefantrine recommends avoiding the following: grapefruit juice; antiarrhythmics, such as amiodarone, disopyramide, flecainide, procainamide and quinidine; antibacterials, such as macrolides and quinolones; all antidepressants; antifungals such as imidazoles and triazoles; terfenadine; other antimalarials; all antipsychotic drugs; and beta blockers, such as metoprolol and sotalol. However, there is no evidence that co-administration with these drugs would be harmful.

A3.8 Primaquine

Molecular weight: 259.4

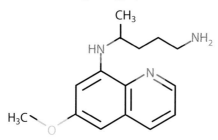

Primaquine is an 8-aminoquinoline and is effective against intrahepatic forms of all types of malaria parasite. It is used to provide radical cure of *P. vivax* and *P. ovale* malaria, in combination with a blood schizontocide for the erythrocytic parasites. Primaquine is also gametocytocidal against *P. falciparum* and has significant blood stage activity against *P. vivax* (and some against asexual stages of *P. falciparum*). The mechanism of action is unknown.

Formulations

• Tablets containing 5.0 mg, 7.5 mg or 15.0 mg of primaquine base as diphosphate.

Pharmacokinetics

Primaquine is readily absorbed from the gastrointestinal tract. Peak plasma concentrations occur around 1–2 h after administration and then decline, with a reported elimination half-life of 3–6 h *(51)*. Primaquine is widely distributed into body tissues. It is rapidly metabolized in the liver. The major metabolite is carboxyprimaquine, which may accumulate in the plasma with repeated administration.

Toxicity

The most important adverse effects are haemolytic anaemia in patients with G6PD deficiency, other defects of the erythrocytic pentose phosphate pathway of glucose metabolism, or some other types of haemoglobinopathy *(52)*. In patients with the African variant of G6PD deficiency, the standard course of primaquine generally produces a benign self-limiting anaemia. In the Mediterranean and Asian variants, haemolysis may be much more severe. Therapeutic doses may also cause abdominal pain if administered on an empty stomach. Larger doses can cause nausea and vomiting. Methaemoglobinaemia may occur. Other uncommon effects include mild anaemia and leukocytosis.

Overdosage may result in leukopenia, agranulocytosis, gastrointestinal symptoms, haemolytic anaemia and methaemoglobinaemia with cyanosis.

Drug interactions

Drugs liable to increase the risk of haemolysis or bone marrow suppression should be avoided.

A3.9 Atovaquone

Molecular weight: 366.8

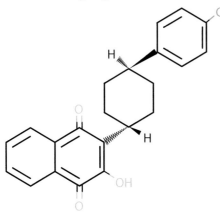

Atovaquone is a hydroxynaphthoquinone antiparasitic drug active against all *Plasmodium* species. It also inhibits pre-erythrocytic development in the liver, and oocyst development in the mosquito. It is combined with proguanil for the treatment of malaria – with which it is synergistic. Atovaquone interferes with cytochrome electron transport.

Formulations

Atovaquone is available for the treatment of malaria in a co-formulation with proguanil:

- Film-coated tablets containing 250 mg of atovaquone and 100 mg of proguanil hydrochloride for adults.
- Tablets containing 62.5 mg of atovaquone and 25 mg of proguanil hydrochloride for paediatric use.

Pharmacokinetics

Atovaquone is poorly absorbed from the gastrointestinal tract but bioavailability following oral administration can be improved by taking the drug with fatty foods. Bioavailabillity is reduced in patients with AIDS. Atovaquone is 99% bound to plasma proteins and has a plasma half-life of around 66–70 h due to enterohepatic recycling. It is excreted almost exclusively in the faeces as unchanged drug. Plasma concentrations are significantly reduced in late pregnancy *(53)*.

Toxicity

Atovaquone is generally very well tolerated *(54)*. Skin rashes, headache, fever, insomnia, nausea, diarrhoea, vomiting, raised liver enzymes, hyponatraemia and, very rarely, haematological disturbances, such as anaemia and neutropenia, have all been reported.

Drug interactions

Reduced plasma concentrations may occur with concomitant administration of metoclopramide, tetracycline and possibly also acyclovir, antidiarrhoeal drugs, benzodiazepines, cephalosporins, laxatives, opioids and paracetamol. Atovaquone decreases the metabolism of zidovudine and cotrimoxazole. Theoretically, it may displace other highly protein-bound drugs from plasma-protein binding sites.

A3.10 Proguanil

Molecular weight: 253.7

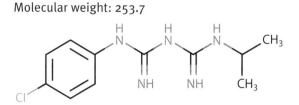

Proguanil is a biguanide compound that is metabolized in the body via the polymorphic cytochrome P450 enzyme CYP2C19 to the active metabolite, cycloguanil. Approximately 3% of Caucasian and African populations and 20% of Oriental people are "poor metabolizers" and have considerably reduced biotransformation of proguanil to cycloguanil *(55, 56)*. Cycloguanil inhibits plasmodial dihydrofolate reductase. The parent compound has weak intrinsic antimalarial activity through an unknown mechanism. It is possibly active against pre-erythrocytic forms of the parasite and is a slow blood schizontocide. Proguanil also has sporontocidal activity, rendering the gametocytes non-infective to the mosquito vector. Proguanil is given as the hydrochloride salt in combination with atovaquone. It is not used alone for treatment as resistance to proguanil develops very quickly. Cycloguanil was formerly administered as an oily suspension of the embonate by intramuscular injection.

Formulations
- Tablets of 100 mg of proguanil hydrochloride containing 87 mg of proguanil base.

In co-formulation with atovaquone:
- Film-coated tablets containing 250 mg of atovaquone and 100 mg of proguanil hydrochloride for adults.
- Tablet containing 62.5 mg of atovaquone and 25 mg of proguanil hydrochloride for paediatric use.

Pharmacokinetics
Proguanil is readily absorbed from the gastrointestinal tract following oral administration. Peak plasma levels occur at about 4 h, and are reduced in the third trimester of pregnancy. Around 75% is bound to plasma proteins. Proguanil is metabolized in the liver to the active antifolate metabolite, cycloguanil, and peak plasma levels of cycloguanil occur 1 h after those of the parent drug. The elimination half-lives of both proguanil and cycloguanil is

approximately 20 h *(57, 58)*. Elimination is about 50% in the urine, of which 60% is unchanged drug and 30% cycloguanil, and a further amount is excreted in the faeces. Small amounts are present in breast milk. The elimination of cycloguanil is determined by that of the parent compound. The biotrans-formation of proguanil to cycloguanil via CYP2C19 is reduced in pregnancy and women taking the oral contraceptive pill *(59, 60)*.

Toxicity

Apart from mild gastric intolerance, diarrhoea, occasional aphthous ulceration and hair loss, there are few adverse effects associated with usual doses of proguanil hydrochloride. Haematological changes (megaloblastic anaemia and pancytopenia) have been reported in patients with severe renal impairment. Overdosage may produce epigastric discomfort, vomiting and haematuria. Proguanil should be used cautiously in patients with renal impairment and the dose reduced according to the degree of impairment.

Drug interactions

Interactions may occur with concomitant administration of warfarin. Absorption of proguanil is reduced with concomitant administration of magnesium trisilicate.

A3.11 Chlorproguanil

Molecular weight: 288.2

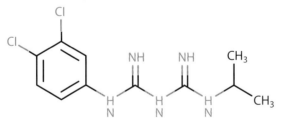

Chlorproguanil is a biguanide and is given as the hydrochloride salt. Its actions and properties are very similar to those of proguanil. It is available only in combination with a sulfone such as dapsone (co-formulated as Lapdap).

Pharmacokinetics

Similar to those of proguanil *(61)*.

Toxicity

As for proguanil.

Drug interactions

As for proguanil.

A3.12 Dapsone

Molecular weight: 248.3

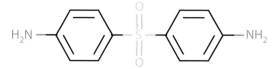

Dapsone is a sulfone widely used for the treatment of leprosy, and sometimes also for treatment or prophylaxis of *Pneumocystis carinii* pneumonia, and treatment of toxoplasmosis, cutaneous leishmaniasis, actinomycetoma and dermatitis herpetiformis. For malaria, dapsone is given in combination with another antimalarial. It is coformulated with chlorproguanil (as Lapdap™). Dapsone inhibits plasmodial dihydropteroate synthase.

Pharmacokinetics

Dapsone is almost completely absorbed from the gastrointestinal tract, with peak plasma concentrations occurring 2–8 h after an oral dose. Dapsone is 50–80% bound to plasma proteins, as is almost 100% of monoacetyldapsone, its major metabolite. Dapsone undergoes enterohepatic recycling. It is widely distributed to body tissues, including breast milk and saliva. Its elimination half-life is 10–50 h. Dapsone is metabolized by acetylation, which exhibits genetic polymorphism. Hydroxylation is the other metabolic pathway, resulting in hydroxylamine dapsone, which may be responsible for dapsone-associated methaemoglobinaemia and haemolysis. Dapsone is mainly excreted in the urine, only 20% as unchanged drug.

Toxicity

Varying degrees of haemolysis and methaemoglobinaemia are the most frequently reported adverse effects and occur in most patients given more than 200 mg of dapsone daily. Doses of up to 100 mg daily do not cause significant haemolysis but patients deficient in G6PD are affected by doses of >50 mg daily. Haemolytic anaemia has been reported following ingestion of dapsone in breast milk. Agranulocytosis has been reported following use of dapsone and pyrimethamine together as malaria prophylaxis – particularly when used twice weekly. Aplastic anaemia has also been reported. Rashes, including pruritus and fixed-drug reactions may occur but serious cutaneous hypersensitivity is rare. "Dapsone syndrome" consists of rash, fever, jaundice and eosinophilia, and has been reported in a few patients using dapsone as malaria prophylaxis, but mainly in leprosy patients on long treatment courses. Other rare adverse effects include anorexia, nausea, vomiting, headache, hepatitis, hypoalbuminaemia and psychosis.

Drug interactions

There is an increased risk of dapsone toxicity with concomitant administration of probenecid, trimethoprim and amprenovir. Levels of dapsone are reduced with rifampicin.

A3.13 Quinine

Molecular weight: 324.4

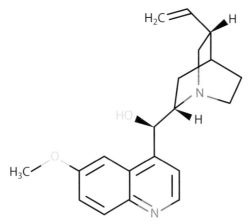

Quinine is an alkaloid derived from the bark of the *Cinchona* tree. Four antimalarial alkaloids can be derived from the bark: quinine (the main alkaloid), quinidine, cinchonine and cinchonidine. Quinine is the L-stereoisomer of quinidine.

Quinine acts principally on the mature trophozoite stage of parasite development and does not prevent sequestration or further development of circulating ring stages of *P. falciparum*. Like other structurally similar antimalarials, quinine also kills the sexual stages of *P. vivax*, *P. malariae* and *P. ovale*, but not mature gametocytes of *P. falciparum*. It does not kill the pre-erythrocytic stages of malaria parasites. The mechanisms of its antimalarial actions are thought to involve inhibition of parasite haem detoxification in the food vacuole, but are not well understood.

Formulations

- Tablets of quinine hydrochloride, quinine dihydrochloride, quinine sulfate and quinine bisulfate containing 82%, 82%, 82.6% and 59.2% quinine base, respectively.
- Injectable solutions of quinine hydrochloride, quinine dihydrochloride and quinine sulfate containing 82%, 82% and 82.6% quinine base, respectively.

Pharmacokinetics

The pharmacokinetic properties of quinine are altered significantly by malaria infection, with reductions in apparent volume of distribution and clearance in proportion to disease severity *(16, 62)*. In children under 2 years of age with severe malaria, concentrations are slightly higher than in older children and adults *(63)*. There is no evidence for dose-dependent kinetics. Quinine is rapidly and almost completely absorbed from the gastrointestinal tract and peak plasma concentrations occur 1–3 h after oral administration of the sulfate or bisulfate *(64)*. It is well absorbed after intramuscular injection in severe malaria *(65, 66)*. Plasma-protein binding, mainly to alpha 1-acid glycoprotein, is 80% in healthy subjects but rises to around 90% in patients with malaria *(67–69)*. Quinine is widely distributed throughout the body including the cerebrospinal fluid (2–7% of plasma values), breast milk (approximate 30% of maternal plasma concentrations) and the placenta *(70)*. Extensive metabolism via the cytochrome P450 enzyme CYP3A4 occurs in the liver and elimination of more polar metabolites is mainly renal *(71, 72)*. The initial metabolite 3-hydroxyquinine contributes approximately 10% of the antimalarial activity of the parent compound, but may accumulate in renal failure *(73)*. Excretion is increased in acid urine. The mean elimination half-life is around 11 h in healthy subjects, 16 h in uncomplicated malaria and 18 h in severe malaria *(62)*. Small amounts appear in the bile and saliva.

Toxicity

Administration of quinine or its salts regularly causes a complex of symptoms known as cinchonism, which is characterized in its mild form by tinnitus, impaired high tone hearing, headache, nausea, dizziness and dysphoria, and sometimes disturbed vision *(7)*. More severe manifestations include vomiting, abdominal pain, diarrhoea and severe vertigo. Hypersensitivity reactions to quinine range from urticaria, bronchospasm, flushing of the skin and fever, through antibody-mediated thrombocytopenia and haemolytic anaemia, to life-threatening haemolytic-uraemic syndrome. Massive haemolysis with renal failure ("black water fever") has been linked epidemiologically and historically to quinine, but its etiology remains uncertain *(74)*. The most important adverse effect in the treatment of severe malaria is hyperinsulinaemic hypoglycaemia *(75)*. This is particularly common in pregnancy (50% of quinine-treated women with severe malaria in late pregnancy). Intramuscular injections of quinine dihydrochloride are acidic (pH 2) and cause pain, focal necrosis and in some cases abscess formation, and in endemic areas are a common cause of sciatic nerve palsy. Hypotension and cardiac arrest may result from rapid intravenous injection. Intravenous quinine should be given only by infusion, never injection. Quinine causes an approximately 10% prolongation of the electrocardiograph QT interval – mainly as a result of slight QRS widening *(75)*. The effect on ventricular repolarization is much less than that with quinidine. Quinine has been used as an abortifacient, but there is no evidence that it causes abortion, premature labour or fetal abnormalities in therapeutic use.

Overdosage of quinine may cause oculotoxicity, including blindness from direct retinal toxicity, and cardiotoxicity, and can be fatal *(76)*. Cardiotoxic effects are less frequent than those of quinidine and include conduction disturbances, arrhythmias, angina, hypotension leading to cardiac arrest and circulatory failure. Treatment is largely supportive, with attention being given to maintenance of blood pressure, glucose and renal function, and to treating arrhythmias.

Drug interactions

There is a theoretical concern that drugs that may prolong the QT interval should not be given with quinine, although whether or not quinine increases the risk of iatrogenic ventricular tachyarrhythmia has not been established. Antiarrhythmics, such as flecainide and amiodarone, should probably be avoided. There might be an increased risk of ventricular arrhythmias with anti-histamines such as terfenadine, and with antipsychotic drugs such as pimozide and thioridazine. Halofantrine, which causes marked QT prolongation, should be avoided but combination with other antimalarials, such as lumefantrine and mefloquine is safe. Quinine increases the plasma concentration of digoxin. Cimetidine inhibits quinine metabolism, causing increased quinine levels and rifampicin increases metabolic clearance leading to low plasma concentrations and an increased therapeutic failure rate (77).

A3.14 Tetracycline

Molecular weight: 444.4

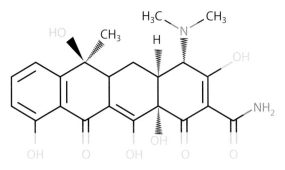

The tetracyclines are a group of antibiotics originally derived from certain *Streptomyces* species, but used mostly in synthetic form. Tetracycline itself may be administered orally or intravenously as the hydrochloride salt or phosphate complex. Both are water soluble, although the intravenous preparation is only stable for a few hours. Tetracyclines are inhibitors of aminoacyl-tRNA binding during protein synthesis. They have a broad range of uses, including treatment of some bacterial infections: *Chlamydia*, *Rickettsia*, *Mycoplasma*, Lyme disease, *Brucella*, tularaemia, plague and cholera. Doxycycline is a synthetic tetracycline with a longer half-life, which makes dosing schedules easier.

Formulations

- Capsules and tablets containing 250 mg of tetracycline hydrochloride, equivalent to 231 mg of tetracycline base.

Pharmacokinetics

Some 60–80% of tetracycline is absorbed from the gastrointestinal tract following oral administration. Absorption is reduced by the presence of divalent and trivalent metal ions with which it forms stable, insoluble complexes. Thus absorption may be impaired with food or milk. Formulation with phosphate may improve absorption. Peak plasma concentrations occur 1–3 h after ingestion. Tetracycline is 20–65% bound to plasma proteins. It is widely distributed throughout the body, although less so than the more lipophilic doxycycline. High concentrations are present in breast milk (around 60% of plasma levels), and also diffuse readily across the placenta, and are retained in sites of new bone formation and teeth development. The half-life of tetracycline is around 8 h;

40–70% is excreted in the urine via glomerular filtration. The remainder is excreted in the faeces and bile. Enterohepatic recycling slows down elimination.

Toxicity

All the tetracyclines have similar adverse effect profiles. Gastrointestinal effects, such as nausea, vomiting and diarrhoea, are common, especially with higher doses, and are due to mucosal irritation. Dry mouth, glossitis, stomatitis, dysphagia and oesophageal ulceration have also been reported. Overgrowth of *Candida* and other bacteria occurs, presumably due to disturbances in gastrointestinal flora as a result of incomplete absorption of the drug. This effect is seen less frequently with doxycycline, which is better absorbed. Pseudomembranous colitis, hepatotoxicity and pancreatitis have also been reported.

Tetracyclines accumulate in patients with renal impairment and this may cause renal failure. In contrast doxycycline accumulates less and is preferred in patient with renal impairment. The use of out-of-date tetracycline can result in the development of a reversible Fanconi-type syndrome characterized by polyuria and polydipsia with nausea, glycosuria, aminoaciduria, hypophos-phataemia, hypokalaemia, and hyperuricaemia with acidosis and proteinuria. These effects have been attributed to the presence of degradation products, in particular anhydroepitetracycline.

Tetracyclines are deposited in deciduous and permanent teeth during their formation and cause discoloration and enamel hypoplasia. They are also deposited in calcifying areas in bone and the nails and interfere with bone growth in young infants or pregnant women. Raised intracranial pressure in adults and infants has also been documented. Tetracyclines use in pregnancy has also been associated with acute fatty liver. Tetracyclines should therefore not be given to pregnant or lactating women, or children of less than 8 years of age.

Hypersensitivity reactions occur, although they are less common than for ß-lactam antibiotics. Rashes, fixed drug reactions, drug fever, angioedema, urticaria, pericarditis and asthma have all been reported. Photosensitivity may develop and, rarely, haemolytic anaemia, eosinophilia, neutropenia and thrombocytopenia. Pre-existing systemic lupus erythematosus may be worsened and tetracyclines are contraindicated in patients with the established disease.

Drug interactions

There is reduced absorption of tetracyclines with concomitant administration of cations, such as aluminium, bismuth, calcium, iron, zinc and magnesium. Administration with antacids, iron preparations, dairy products and some other foods should therefore be avoided. Nephrotoxicity may be exacerbated with diuretics, methoxyflurane or other potentially nephrotoxic drugs. Potentially hepatotoxic drugs should be avoided. Tetracyclines produce increased concentrations of digoxin, lithium and theophylline, and decrease plasma atovaquone concentrations and also the effectiveness of oral contraceptives. They may antagonize the actions of penicillins so should not be given concomitantly.

A3.15 Doxycycline

(See also tetracycline)
Molecular weight: 444.4

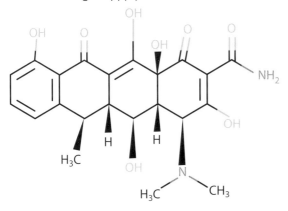

Doxycycline is a tetracycline derivative with uses similar to those of tetracycline. It may be preferred to tetracycline because of its longer half-life, more reliable absorption and better safety profile in patients with renal insufficiency, where it may be used with caution. It is relatively water insoluble but very lipid soluble. It may be given orally or intravenously. It is available as the hydrochloride salt or phosphate complex, or as a complex prepared from the hydrochloride and calcium chloride.

Formulations

● Capsules and tablets containing 100 mg of doxycycline salt as hydrochloride.

Pharmacokinetics

Doxycycline is readily and almost completely absorbed from the gastrointestinal tract and absorption is not affected significantly by the presence of food. Peak plasma concentrations occur 2 h after administration. Some 80–95% is protein-bound and half-life is 10–24 h *(78)*. It is widely distributed in body tissues and fluids. In patients with normal renal function, 40% of doxycycline is excreted in the urine, although more if the urine is alkalinized. It may accumulate in renal failure. However, the majority of the dose is excreted in the faeces.

Toxicity

As for tetracycline. Gastrointestinal effects are fewer than with tetracycline, although oesophageal ulceration can still be a problem if insufficient water is taken with tablets or capsules. There is less accumulation in patients with renal impairment. Doxycycline should not be given to pregnant or lactating women, or children aged up to 8 years.

Drug interactions

Doxycycline has a lower affinity for binding with calcium than other tetracyclines, so may be taken with food or milk. However, antacids and iron may still affect absorption. Metabolism may be accelerated by drugs that induce hepatic enzymes, such as carbamazepine, phenytoin, phenobarbital and rifampicin, and by chronic alcohol use.

A3.16 Clindamycin

Molecular weight: 425.0

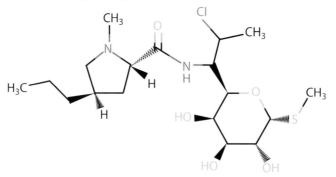

Clindamycin is a lincosamide antibiotic, i.e. a chlorinated derivative of lincomycin. It is very soluble in water. It inhibits the early stages of protein synthesis by a mechanism similar to that of the macrolides. It may be administered by mouth as capsules containing the hydrochloride or as oral liquid preparations containing the palmitate hydrochloride. Clindamycin is given parenterally as the phosphate either by the intramuscular or the intravenous route. It is used for the treatment of anaerobic and Gram-positive bacterial infections, babesiosis, toxoplasmosis and *Pneumocystis carinii* pneumonia.

Formulations

- Capsules containing 75 mg, 150 mg or 300 mg of clindamycin base as hydrochloride.

Pharmacokinetics

About 90% of a dose is absorbed following oral administration. Food does not impede absorption but may delay it. Clindamycin phosphate and palmitate hydrochloride are rapidly hydrolysed to form the free drug. Peak concentrations may be reached within 1 h in children and 3 h in adults. It is widely distributed, although not into the cerebrospinal fluid. It crosses the placenta and appears in breast milk. It is 90% bound to plasma proteins and accumulates in leukocytes, macrophages and bile. The half-life is 2–3 h but this may be prolonged in neonates and patients with renal impairment. Clindamycin undergoes metabolism to the active *N*-demethyl and sulfoxide metabolites, and also some inactive metabolites. About 10% of a dose is excreted in the urine as active drug or metabolites and about 4% in the faeces. The remainder is excreted as inactive metabolites. Excretion is slow and takes place over many days. Clindamycin is not effectively removed from the body by dialysis.

Toxicity

Diarrhoea occurs in 2–20% of patients. In some, pseudomembranous colitis may develop during or after treatment, which can be fatal. Other reported gastro-intestinal effects include nausea, vomiting, abdominal pain and an unpleasant taste in the mouth. Around 10% of patients develop a hypersensitivity reaction. This may take the form of skin rash, urticaria or anaphylaxis. Other adverse effects include leukopenia, agranulocytosis, eosinophilia, thrombocytopenia, erythema multiforme, polyarthritis, jaundice and hepatic damage. Some parenteral formulations contain benzyl alcohol, which may cause fatal "gasping syndrome" in neonates.

Drug interactions

Clindamycin may enhance the effects of drugs with neuromuscular blocking activity and there is a potential danger of respiratory depression. Additive respiratory depressant effects may also occur with opioids. Clindamycin may antagonize the activity of parasympathomimetics.

A3.17 Pharmacology of antimalarials in special groups and conditions

A3.17.1 Safety and tolerability of antimalarials in infants

Infants under 12 months of age constitute a significant proportion of patients in malaria endemic countries. Yet few studies focus specifically on this age range, partly because of ethical dilemmas and also owing to technical difficulties with sampling. Very young children cannot report adverse effects themselves, so detection of these is dependent upon parents and health professionals making observations. In addition, pre-marketing clinical trials for new drugs are not represented by important subpopulations including infants *(79)*, yet there are potentially important pharmacokinetic differences in infants compared to older children and adults *(80)*.

Drug absorption

The gastric pH at birth is usually 6–8 but within a few hours falls to 2 and then rises again until virtual achlorhydria occurs for several days. As the gastric mucosa develops, the acidity increases again until 3 years of age when adult values are attained. The gastric emptying time is prolonged (up to 8 h) in neonates and approaches adult values only after 6 months. Intramuscular injections can also be problematic in young children. Infants with acute or severe malaria may become extremely "shut down" whereby visceral, muscle and skin blood flow is reduced. This may result in slow, erratic or incomplete drug absorption and the consequent delay in achieving therapeutic drug levels at a time when speed and adequacy of drug delivery are crucial.

Distribution

Relatively large total and extracellular body water compartments in infancy lead to larger apparent volumes of distribution. Total body lipids rise steadily after birth for the first 9 months of life but then decrease until adolescence. These changes in body composition can modulate volume of distribution and clearance. Liver mass per body weight is higher in infants than adults and the liver undergoes rapid growth during the first 2 years. The brain is dispropor-tionately large in young children, and the blood brain barrier relatively immature, making a further contribution to volume of distribution. Finally drug distribution is also affected by lower protein binding in infancy with more free drug and thus increased clearance. The former might also lead to a greater risk of toxicity.

Drug metabolism

The cytochrome P450 mixed function oxidase system is the most important biotransformation system incorporating many enzymes and isoenzymes. In general, these enzyme systems are immature at birth. There is therefore relatively slow clearance of most metabolized drugs in the first 2–3 months of life. Between 2 and 6 months clearance is more rapid than in adults and even more so for most drugs from 6 months to 2 years (elimination half-life for metabolized drugs in infants aged 6 months to 2 years is 0.6 times that in adults).

Renal clearance

Glomerular filtration rate only reaches surface-area-adjusted adult levels at around 6 months of age. Thus for drugs that rely on renal elimination, elimination half-lives in very young infants may be up to 2–3 times longer than in adults. After 2 months, half-lives are shorter (0.35–0.5 times adult values) until about 2 years of age.

A3.17.2 Malnutrition and antimalarials

Malaria and malnutrition frequently coexist. The relationship between malaria and nutritional status is complex and has been the subject of debate for many years *(81)*. Given that a significant proportion of the world's malnourished children live in malaria endemic countries *(82)* it is important to understand how antimalarial drug disposition may be affected when malnutrition is severe. This section outlines the physiological changes that occur in malnourished patients and discusses how these may influence the pharmacokinetic properties of antimalarials, drawing on the few studies of antimalarial drug disposition in malnutrition that are available

Note: in reviewing the literature it was apparent that many studies were conducted in populations and settings where some degree of malnutrition would have been expected. However, this was only rarely mentioned as a possible confounder for drug efficacy, although there was an occasional comment that obviously malnourished patients appeared to respond differently to treatment than did other patients *(83)*. Several ongoing studies are planning to look specifically at treatment outcomes in this group of patients.

Definitions

There are different ways of classifying malnutrition. Earlier studies employ the Wellcome classification: where body weight is given as a percentage of standard weight (50th percentile of the Harvard value): underweight 80–60%; marasmus 60%; kwashiorkor 80–60% + oedema; marasmic kwashiorkor 60% + oedema. Other studies refer to low weight-for-height (wasting); low weight-for-age (underweight); or low height-for-age (stunting) and use anthropometric indicators and reference standards. Protein-energy malnutrition is defined as a range of pathological conditions arising from coincident lack, in varying proportions, of protein and calories, occurring most frequently in infants and young children and commonly associated with infections *(84)*.

Pharmacokinetics

Absorption

Anorexia, diarrhoea and vomiting are common. Anorexia will affect the absorption of drugs requiring concomitant administration of fatty foods, and oral bioavailability will be reduced in vomiting patients or those with a rapid transit time. Atrophy of the bowel mucosa, which occurs in severe protein-energy malnutrition, will also hinder absorption.

Children with oedematous lower limbs may be expected to have altered absorption from intramuscular injections. Patients with protein-energy malnutrition frequently have poor peripheral perfusion due to circulatory insufficiency associated with bradycardia, hypotension and a reduced cardiac output. Thus absorption of intramuscular and possibly intrarectal drugs may be expected to be slower than in patients without protein-energy malnutrition. Diminished muscle mass may make repeated intramuscular injections difficult.

Distribution

Total body water increases in proportion to the degree of malnutrition, mainly owing to an expansion of the extracellular fluid (most obvious in oedematous patients). Thus the volume of distribution of some drugs can be expected to be larger and plasma concentrations lower. Albumin is the most important plasma protein for binding of many drugs, but in protein-energy malnutrition hypoalbuminaemia results from decreased synthesis as dietary deficiency occurs. With highly bound drugs this could in theory lead to an increase in the amount of unbound drug, which may increase both the elimination, since more drug is available for metabolism, and potential toxicity. There are other plasma proteins less severely affected by decreased synthesis, and if these are able to bind some free drug, then the increase in free fraction might not be as great as anticipated.

Metabolism

Fatty infiltration occurs but jaundice is uncommon unless septicaemia is present. Liver function tests may be abnormal and urea cycle enzymes are decreased. Children with kwashiorkor excreted a higher proportion of unchanged chloroquine before therapy than in the recovery phase *(85)*. This suggests that hepatic function was inadequate during the acute phase of kwashiorkor. Animal studies have demonstrated that some enzyme systems, such as cytochrome P450, have decreased activity in the presence of significant malnutrition.

Elimination

Owing to the reduction in cardiac output, the kidneys receive less than the usual 25% of renal blood flow. Glomerular filtration rate, renal blood flow and tubular function have all been shown to be inadequate, and compounded by concomitant dehydration. Drugs dependent on renal excretion might be expected to have elevated plasma concentrations under such circumstances. Abnormal excretion of drugs into bile has also been described in severe protein-energy malnutrition.

Antimalarials and protein-energy malnutrition

Chloroquine

Few data are available for chloroquine kinetics in malnourished patients. Children with kwashiorkor excreted a higher ratio of chloroquine to its metabolites before nutritional rehabilitation *(85)*. Presumably the metabolism of chloroquine by the liver was affected adversely in protein-energy malnutrition. In a study of chloroquine pharmacokinetics in five children with kwashiorkor (but without malaria), peak plasma concentrations of the drug were approximately one-third of the values for healthy controls (mean 40 + 30 ng/ml compared to 134 + 99 ng/ml), but the times to peak levels and the elimination half-lives were not significantly different, indicating reduced absorption. There was also reduced metabolism of chloroquine to its metabolite, desethyl-chloroquine, which suggested some impairment of drug metabolism. However, the study did not consider plasma protein binding or drug distribution. Currently there are no recommendations for dose alterations in patients with protein-energy malnutrition *(86)*.

Quinine

Three studies examining the kinetics of quinine in malnourished patients have been published. The first from Nigeria compared the pharmacokinetics of an oral dose of quinine 10 mg/kg in six children with kwashiorkor and seven normal controls who were attending a malaria follow-up clinic *(87)*. The children were aged 1–3 years. Values for total plasma proteins and albumin for children with kwashiorkor were 74% and 67% of those for control children. Absorption of quinine was slower in the kwashiorkor group than in the controls (mean time to maximum concentration (t_{max}) 2.5 ± 0.3 h compared to 1.5 ± 0.6 h);

maximum plasma concentration (C_{max}) was also lower (1.7 ± 0.5 µmol/l compared to 2.4 + 0.3 µmol/l). Rate of clearance of quinine in kwashiorkor was less than one-third of the value for well-nourished patients (31.5 ± 8.5 mg/min compared to 108.5 ± 34.8 mg/min) and the elimination half-life was also longer (15.0 ± 4.4 h compared to 8.0 ± 1.3 h). The authors concluded that the combination of malabsorption, reduced plasma protein binding and reduced metabolism in the liver was responsible for the differences observed. No dose alterations were suggested.

The second study, in Gabon, compared eight children with non-kwashiorkor global malnutrition (defined as having a ratio of left mid-arm circumference:head circumference < 0.279) with seven children with normal nutritional status *(88)*. The children were aged 9–60 months. Only two were subsequently confirmed to have malaria, although all had been febrile at presentation. Mean serum albumin levels in the two groups were 28.7 and 31.0 respectively. Each child received a loading dose of 16 mg/kg quinine base (25 mg/kg quinine resorcine hydrochloride; Quinimax) by deep intramuscular injection followed by 8 mg/kg at 12 h. The t_{max} was significantly shorter in malnourished children (1.1 ± 0.4 h compared to 2.2 ± 1.2 h). No difference was observed for C_{max}, volume of distribution or protein binding. Clearance was significantly faster for malnourished children (4.4 ± 3.6 ml/min/kg compared to 2.3 ± 1.4 ml/min/kg), and half-life shorter (6.3 ± 1.8 h compared to 10.1 ± 3.4 h). Concentration at 12 h was lower in malnourished children (3.3 ± 1.6 mg/ml compared to 5.3 ± 1.6 mg/l). There was a significant correlation between elimination half-life and left mid-arm:head circumference. The ratio between the area under the curve for hydroxyquinine, the main metabolite of quinine, and that for quinine was significantly higher in the malnourished group and significantly correlated with left mid-arm:head circumference ratio, indicating increased metabolism of quinine in malnourished patients. The authors suggest that the administration interval should be reduced to 8 h in malnourished children in order to obtain plasma concentrations of quinine similar to those found in children with normal nutrition.

In the third study, from Niger, 40 children were divided into four groups: normally nourished children with or without cerebral malaria, and malnourished children (>2 SD below the median value for at least two of the following: weight-for-height, weight-for-age and height-for-age) with or without cerebral malaria *(89)*. The age range studied was 24–72 months. Patients with kwashiorkor were excluded. All patients received 4.7 mg/kg quinine base (as 8 mg/kg Quinimax) by intravenous infusion over 4 h. Infusions were repeated every 8 h for children with cerebral malaria. C_{max} was highest in malnourished children, and was higher in those without malaria than with malaria (8.5 ± 4.7 mg/l compared to 7.7 ± 2.0 mg/l); it was lowest in the control groups without and with malaria

(3.0 ± 2.1 mg/l and 6.6 ± 3.0 mg/l). There were no differences between the area under the curve for 0—8 h and elimination half-life for the two malnutrition groups and controls with malaria, but all were higher than for controls without malaria. Conversely plasma clearance of quinine and volume of distribution were smaller in these three groups than in controls without malaria. Alpha 1-glycoprotein plasma concentrations and protein-bound fraction of the drug were increased in the three groups. Malnourished children had slower parasite clearance but the difference was not significant. The authors concluded that severe global malnutrition and cerebral malaria have a similar effect on quinine pharmacokinetics in children and that cerebral malaria-mediated modifications of quinine disposition are not potentiated. They recommend that current dosing schedules should not be altered for children with malnutrition.

Sulfadoxine-pyrimethamine

No studies exist of sulfadoxine-pyrimethamine kinetics in malnourished patients. However, observational data from Rwandan refugee children showed that malnourished children (defined as weight-for-height < 80% of the reference median with or without oedema) were more likely to have treatment failure than children without malnutrition (86% compared to 58% (83). Higher initial parasite counts and host immunity, as well as pharmacokinetic differences, may also have contributed to this finding.

Tetracycline

A number of small studies have been conducted on tetracycline kinetics in malnourished adults from India. One study compared the kinetics of intravenous and oral tetracycline in malnourished and normal adult males (90). Compared to the control group, malnourished patients had lower protein binding, shorter elimination half-life and reduced volume of distribution. The authors suggest that in order to keep levels of tetracycline above the minimum inhibitory concentration, the dose interval should be reduced. A similar conclusion was reached by another study that also found more rapid distribution of tetracycline and faster clearance in the malnourished group (91). The same author, in a separate study, also looked at absorption of oral compared with intravenous tetracycline in various types of malnutrition. Oral absorption was slower in patients with protein-energy-malnutrition and pellagra than in patients with anaemia or vitamin B complex deficiency patients and healthy controls. In a third study, patients with nutritional oedema were found to have increased C_{max} and area under the curve values, and reduced clearance and volume of distribution compared with healthy controls (i.e. some differences with non-oedema malnutrition patients) (92).

Doxycycline

There is a single study examining the kinetics of doxycycline given orally to adult patients in India *(93)*. Area under the curve, elimination half-life and plasma protein binding were reduced, and clearance increased in the malnourished group. Renal clearance was similar in controls and malnourished patients. The authors surmised that increased total body clearance of doxycycline might be due to higher metabolism in malnourished patients. Steady state plasma C_{min} levels were lower than in healthy patients but still within the therapeutic range. A change in dose recommendation does not seem necessary given these findings.

Other antimalarials

There are no studies of the kinetics of clindamycin, amodiaquine, artemisinin derivatives (dihydroartemisinin), artemether-lumefantrine, mefloquine or primaquine kinetics in malnourished patients.

Conclusion

There are many reasons why pharmacokinetics may be different in malnourished patients compared to those who are well nourished. However, with the possible exception of quinine, there are insufficient data available for specific dosing changes to be recommended.

A3.18 References[24]

1. Krugliak M, Ginsburg H. Studies on the antimalarial mode of action of quinoline-containing drugs: time-dependence and irreversibility of drug action, and interactions with compounds that alter the function of the parasite's food vacuole. *Life Sciences*, 1991, 49:1213–1219.

2. Bray PG et al. Access to hematin: the basis of chloroquine resistance. *Molecular Pharmacology*, 1998, 54:170–179.

3. Gustafsson LL et al. Disposition of chloroquine in man after single intravenous and oral doses. *British Journal of Clinical Pharmacology*, 1983, 15:471–479.

4. Walker O et al. Plasma chloroquine and desethylchloroquine concentrations in children during and after chloroquine treatment for malaria. *British Journal of Clinical Pharmacology*, 1983:16:701–705.

---

[24] Further information on the chemistry and pharmacology of antimalarials can be obtained from the web site of the United States National Library of Medicines, Specialized Information Services, ChemIDplus Advanced: http://chem.sis.nlm.nih.gov/chemidplus.

5. White NJ et al. Chloroquine treatment of severe malaria in children. Pharmacokinetics, toxicity, and new dosage recommendations. *New England Journal of Medicine*, 1988, 319:1493–1500.

6. Mnyika KS, Kihamia CM. Chloroquine-induced pruritus: its impact on chloroquine utilization in malaria control in Dar es Salaam. *Journal of Tropical Medicine and Hygiene*, 1991, 94:27–31.

7. Taylor WR, White NJ. Antimalarial drug toxicity: a review. *Drug Safety*, 2004, 27:25–61.

8. Riou B et al. Treatment of severe chloroquine poisoning. *New England Journal of Medicine*, 1988, 318:1–6.

9. Clemessy JL et al. Treatment of acute chloroquine poisoning: a 5-year experience. *Critical Care Medicine*, 1996, 24:1189–1195.

10. Winstanley PA et al. The disposition of amodiaquine in Zambians and Nigerians with malaria. *British Journal of Clinical Pharmacology*, 1990, 29:695–701.

11. Hatton CS et al. Frequency of severe neutropenia associated with amodiaquine prophylaxis against malaria. *Lancet*, 1986, 1:411–414.

12. Miller KD et al. Severe cutaneous reactions among American travelers using pyrimethamine-sulfadoxine (Fansidar) for malaria prophylaxis. *American Journal of Tropical Medicine and Hygiene*, 1986, 35:451–458.

13. Bjorkman A, Phillips-Howard PA. Adverse reactions to sulfa drugs: implications for malaria chemotherapy. *Bulletin of the World Health Organization*, 1991, 69:297–304.

14. Winstanley PA et al. The disposition of oral and intramuscular pyrimethamine/sulphadoxine in Kenyan children with high parasitaemia but clinically non-severe falciparum malaria. *British Journal of Clinical Pharmacology*, 1992, 33:143–148.

15. Price R et al. Pharmacokinetics of mefloquine combined with artesunate in children with acute falciparum malaria. *Antimicrobial Agents and Chemotherapy*, 1999, 43:341–346.

16. Krishna S, White NJ. Pharmacokinetics of quinine, chloroquine and amodiaquine. Clinical implications. *Clinical Pharmacokinetics*, 1996, 30:263–299

17. Simpson JA et al. Population pharmacokinetics of mefloquine in patients with acute falciparum malaria. *Clinical Pharmacology and Therapeutics*, 1999, 66:472–484.

18. Slutsker LM et al. Mefloquine therapy for *Plasmodium falciparum* malaria in children under 5 years of age in Malawi: in vivo/in vitro efficacy and correlation of drug concentration with parasitological outcome. *Bulletin of the World Health Organization*, 1990, 68:53–59.

19. Karbwang J et al. Pharmacokinetics and pharmacodynamics of mefloquine in Thai patients with acute falciparum malaria. *Bulletin of the World Health Organization*, 1991, 69:207–212.

20. Nosten F et al. Mefloquine pharmacokinetics and resistance in children with acute falciparum malaria. *British Journal of Clinical Pharmacology*, 1991, 31:556–559.

21. Svensson US et al. Population pharmacokinetic and pharmacodynamic modelling of artemisinin and mefloquine enantiomers in patients with falciparum malaria. *European Journal of Clinical Pharmacology*, 2002, 58:339–351.

22. Gimenez F et al. Stereoselective pharmacokinetics of mefloquine in healthy Caucasians after multiple doses. *Journal of Pharmaceutical Sciences*, 1994, 83:824–827.

23. Bourahla A et al. Stereoselective pharmacokinetics of mefloquine in young children. *European Journal of Clinical Pharmacology*, 1996, 50:241–244.

24. Bem JL, Kerr L, Stuerchler D. Mefloquine prophylaxis: an overview of spontaneous reports of severe psychiatric reactions and convulsions. *Journal of Tropical Medicine and Hygiene*, 1992, 95:167–179.

25. ter Kuile FO et al. Mefloquine treatment of acute falciparum malaria: a prospective study of non-serious adverse effects in 3673 patients. *Bulletin of the World Health Organization*, 1995, 73:631–642.

26. Phillips-Howard PA, ter Kuile FO. CNS adverse events associated with antimalarial agents. Fact or fiction? *Drug Safety*, 1995, 12:370–383.

27. Mai NTH et al. Post-malaria neurological syndrome. *Lancet*, 1996, 348:917–921.

28. Supanaranond W et al. Lack of a significant adverse cardiovascular effect of combined quinine and mefloquine therapy for uncomplicated malaria. *Transactions of the Royal Society of Tropical Medicine and Hygiene*, 1997, 91:694–696.

29. Eckstein-Ludwig U et al. Artemisinins target the SERCA of *Plasmodium falciparum*. *Nature*, 2003, 424:957–961.

30. Navaratnam V et al. Pharmacokinetics of artemisinin-type compounds. *Clinical Pharmacokinetics*, 2000, 39:255–270.

31. Ashton M, Nguyen DS, Nguyen VH, et al. Artemisinin kinetics and dynamics during oral and rectal treatment of uncomplicated malaria. *Clinical Pharmacology and Therapeutics*, 1998, 63:482–493.

32. Ribeiro IR, Olliaro P. Safety of artemisinin and its derivatives. A review of published and unpublished clinical trials. *Medicine Tropical (Mars)*, 1998, 58(3 Suppl.):50–53.

33. Price R et al. Adverse effects in patients with acute falciparum malaria treated with artemisinin derivatives. *American Journal of Tropical Medicine and Hygiene*, 1999, 60:547–555.

34. Leonardi E et al. Severe allergic reactions to oral artesunate: a report of two cases. *Transactions of the Royal Society of Tropical Medicine and Hygiene*, 2001, 95:182–183.

35. van Vugt M et al. A case-control auditory evaluation of patients treated with artemisinin derivatives for multidrug-resistant *Plasmodium falciparum* malaria. *American Journal of Tropical Medicine and Hygiene*, 2000, 62:65–69.

36. Kissinger E et al. Clinical and neurophysiological study of the effects of multiple doses of artemisinin on brain-stem function in Vietnamese patients. *American Journal of Tropical Medicine and Hygiene*, 2000, 63:48–55.

37. Hien TT et al. Neuropathological assessment of artemether-treated severe malaria. *Lancet*, 2003, 362:295–296.

37[a] *Assessment of the safety of artemisinin compounds in pregnancy.* Geneva, World Health Organization, 2003 (document WHO/CDS/MAL/2003.1094).

38. Ezzet F, Mull R, Karbwang J. Population pharmacokinetics and therapeutic response of CGP 56697 (artemether + benflumetol) in malaria patients. *British Journal of Clinical Pharmacology*, 1998, 46:553–561.

39. Murphy SA et al. The disposition of intramuscular artemether in children with cerebral malaria; a preliminary study. *Transactions of the Royal Society of Tropical Medicine and Hygiene*, 1997, 91:331–334.

40. Hien TT et al. Comparative pharmacokinetics of intramuscular artesunate and artemether in patients with severe falciparum malaria. *Antimicrobial Agents and Chemotherapy*, 2004, 48:4234–4239.

41. Mithwani S et al. Population pharmacokinetics of artemether and dihydro-artemisinin following single intramuscular dosing of artemether in African children with severe falciparum malaria. *British Journal of Clinical Pharmacology*, 2004, 57:146–152.

42. Brewer TG et al. Neurotoxicity in animals due to arteether and artemether. *Transactions of the Royal Society of Tropical Medicine and Hygiene*, 1994, 88 (Suppl. 1):S33–36.

43. Bethell DB et al. Pharmacokinetics of oral artesunate in children with moderately severe *Plasmodium falciparum* malaria. *Transactions of the Royal Society of Tropical Medicine and Hygiene*, 1997, 91:195–198.

44. Batty KT et al. A pharmacokinetic and pharmacodynamic study of intravenous vs oral artesunate in uncomplicated falciparum malaria. *British Journal of Clinical Pharmacology*, 1998, 45:123–129.

45. Newton PN et al. Antimalarial bioavailability and disposition of artesunate in acute falciparum malaria. *Antimicrobial Agents and Chemotherapy*, 2000, 44:972–997.

46. Krishna S et al. Bioavailability and preliminary clinical efficacy of intrarectal artesunate in Ghanaian children with moderate malaria. *Antimicrobial Agents and Chemotherapy*, 2001, 45:509–516.

47. Ilett KF et al. The pharmacokinetic properties of intramuscular artesunate and rectal dihydroartemisinin in uncomplicated falciparum malaria. *British Journal of Clinical Pharmacology*, 2002, 53:23–30.

48. Newton PN et al. Comparison of oral artesunate and dihydroartemisinin antimalarial bioavailabilities in acute falciparum malaria. *Antimicrobial Agents and Chemotherapy*, 2002, 46:1125–1127.

49. White NJ, van Vugt M, Ezzet F. Clinical pharmacokinetics and pharmacodynamics of artemether-lumefantrine. *Clinical Pharmacokinetics*, 1999, 37:105–125.

50. van Vugt M et al. No evidence of cardiotoxicity during antimalarial treatment with artemether-lumefantrine. *American Journal of Tropical Medicine and Hygiene*, 1999, 61:964–967.

51. Mihaly GW et al. Pharmacokinetics of primaquine in man: identification of the carboxylic acid derivative as a major plasma metabolite. *British Journal of Clinical Pharmacology*, 1984, 17:441–446.

52. Chan TK, Todd D, Tso SC. Drug-induced haemolysis in glucose-6-phosphate dehydrogenase deficiency. *British Medical Journal*, 1976, 2:1227–1229.

53. McGready R et al. The pharmacokinetics of atovaquone and proguanil in pregnant women with acute falciparum malaria. *European Journal of Clinical Pharmacology*, 2003, 59:545–552.

54. Sabchareon A et al. Efficacy and pharmacokinetics of atovaquone and proguanil in children with multidrug-resistant *Plasmodium falciparum* malaria. *Transactions of the Royal Society of Tropical Medicine and Hygiene*, 1998, 92:201–206.

55. Helsby NA et al. The pharmacokinetics and activation of proguanil in man: consequences of variability in drug metabolism. *British Journal of Clinical Pharmacology*, 1990, 30:593–598.

56. Kaneko A et al. Proguanil disposition and toxicity in malaria patients from Vanuatu with high frequencies of CYP2C19 mutations. *Pharmacogenetics*, 1999, 9:317–326.

57. Wattanagoon Y et al. Single dose pharmacokinetics of proguanil and its metabolites in healthy subjects. *British Journal of Clinical Pharmacology*, 1987, 24:775–780.

58. Hussein Z et al. Population pharmacokinetics of proguanil in patients with acute *P. falciparum* malaria after combined therapy with atovaquone. *British Journal of Clinical Pharmacology*, 1996, 42:589–597.

59. Wangboonskul J et al. Single dose pharmacokinetics of proguanil and its metabolites in pregnancy. *European Journal of Clinical Pharmacology*, 1993, 44:247–251.

60. McGready R et al. Pregnancy and use of oral contraceptives reduces the biotransformation of proguanil to cycloguanil. *European Journal of Clinical Pharmacology*, 2003, 59:553–557.

61. Veenendaal JR, Edstein MD, Rieckmann KH. Pharmacokinetics of chlorproguanil in man after a single oral dose of Lapudrine. *Chemotherapy*, 1988, 34:275–283.

62. White NJ et al. Quinine pharmacokinetics and toxicity in cerebral and uncomplicated falciparum malaria. *American Journal of Medicine*, 1982, 73:564–572.

63. van Hensbroek MB et al. Quinine pharmacokinetics in young children with severe malaria. *American Journal of Tropical Medicine and Hygiene*, 1996, 54:237–242.

64. Supanaranond W et al. Disposition of oral quinine in acute falciparum malaria. *European Journal of Clinical Pharmacology*, 1991, 40:49–52.

65. Waller D et al. The pharmacokinetic properties of intramuscular quinine in Gambian children with severe falciparum malaria. *Transactions of the Royal Society of Tropical Medicine and Hygiene*, 1990. 84:488–491.

66. White NJ. Optimal regimens of parenteral quinine. *Transactions of the Royal Society of Tropical Medicine and Hygiene*, 1995, 89:462–464.

67. Silamut K et al. Binding of quinine to plasma proteins in falciparum malaria. *American Journal of Tropical Medicine and Hygiene*, 1985, 34:681–686.

68. Silamut K et al. Alpha 1-acid glycoprotein (orosomucoid) and plasma protein binding of quinine in falciparum malaria. *British Journal of Clinical Pharmacology*, 1991, 32:311–315.

69. Mansor SM et al. Effect of *Plasmodium falciparum* malaria infection on the plasma concentration of alpha 1-acid glycoprotein and the binding of quinine in Malawian children. *British Journal of Clinical Pharmacology*, 1991, 32:317–321.

70. Phillips RE et al. Quinine pharmacokinetics and toxicity in pregnant and lactating women with falciparum malaria. *British Journal of Clinical Pharmacology*, 1986, 21:677–683.

71. Hall AP et al. Human plasma and urine quinine levels following tablets, capsules, and intravenous infusion. *Clinical Pharmacology and Therapeutics*, 1973, 14:580–585.

72. Pukrittayakamee S et al. A study of the factors affecting the metabolic clearance of quinine in malaria. *European Journal of Clinical Pharmacology*, 1997, 52:487–493.

73. Newton PN et al. Pharmacokinetics of quinine and 3-hydroxyquinine in severe falciparum malaria with acute renal failure. *Transactions of the Royal Society of Tropical Medicine and Hygiene*, 1999, 93:69–72.

74. Bruce-Chwatt LJ. Quinine and the mystery of blackwater fever. *Acta Leidensia*, 1987, 55:181–196.

75. White NJ, Looareesuwan S, Warrell DA. Quinine and quinidine: a comparison of EKG effects during the treatment of malaria. *Journal of Cardiovascular Pharmacology*, 1983, 5:173–175.

76. Boland ME, Roper SM, Henry JA. Complications of quinine poisoning. *Lancet*, 1985, 1:384–385.

77. Pukrittayakamee S et al. Adverse effect of rifampicin on quinine efficacy in uncomplicated falciparum malaria. *Antimicrobial Agents and Chemotherapy*, 2003, 47:1509-1513.

78. Newton PN et al. The Pharmacokinetics of oral doxycycline during combination treatment of severe falciparum malaria. *Antimicrobial Agents and Chemotherapy*, 2005, 49:1622–1625.

79. Atuah KN, Hughes D, Pirmohamed M. Clinical pharmacology: special safety considerations in drug development and pharmacovigilance. *Drug Safety*, 2004, 27:535–554.

80. Ginsberg G et al. Pediatric pharmacokinetic data: implications for environmental risk assessment for children. *Pediatrics*, 2004, 113(4 Suppl.):973–983.

81. Shankar AH. Nutritional modulation of malaria morbidity and mortality. *Journal of Infectious Diseases*, 2000, 182(Suppl. 1):S37–S53.

82. de Onis M et al. The worldwide magnitude of protein-energy malnutrition: an overview from the WHO Global Database on Child Growth. *Bulletin of the World Health Organization*, 1993, 71:703–712.

83. Wolday D et al. Sensitivity of *Plasmodium falciparum in vivo* to chloroquine and pyrimethamine-sulfadoxine in Rwandan patients in a refugee camp in Zaire. *Transactions of the Royal Society of Tropical Medicine and Hygiene*, 1995, 89:654–656.

84. Wellcome Trust Working Party. Classification of infantile malnutrition. *Lancet*, 1970, 2:302–303.

85. Wharton BA, McChesney EW. Chloroquine metabolism in kwashiorkor. *Journal of Tropical Pediatrics*, 1970, 16:130–132.

86. Walker O et al. Single dose disposition of chloroquine in kwashiorkor and normal children – evidence for decreased absorption in kwashiorkor. *British Journal of Clinical Pharmacology*, 1987, 23:467–472.

87. Salako LA, Sowunmi A, Akinbami FO. Pharmacokinetics of quinine in African children suffering from kwashiorkor. *British Journal of Clinical Pharmacology*, 1989, 28:197–201.

88. Treluyer JM et al. Metabolism of quinine in children with global malnutrition. *Pediatric Research*, 1996, 40:558–563.

89. Pussard E et al. Quinine disposition in globally malnourished children with cerebral malaria. *Clinical Pharmacology and Therapeutics*, 1999, 65:500–510.

90. Shastri RA, Krishnaswamy K. Undernutrition and tetracycline half life. *Clinica Chimica Acta*, 1976 66:157–164.

91. Raghuram TC, Krishnaswamy K. Tetracycline kinetics in undernourished subjects. *International Journal of Clinical Pharmacology, Therapy, and Toxicology*, 1981, 19:409–413.

92. Raghuram TC, Krishnaswamy K. Tetracycline absorption in malnutrition. *Drug-Nutrition Interactions*, 1981, 1:23–29.

93. Raghuram TC, Krishnaswamy K. Pharmacokinetics and plasma steady state levels of doxycycline in undernutrition. *British Journal of Clinical Pharmacology*, 1982, 14:785–789.

ANNEX 4

ANTIMALARIALS AND MALARIA TRANSMISSION

A4.1 Principles of malaria transmission

Malaria is spread from person to person by mosquitoes belonging to the genus *Anopheles*. The female mosquito is infected by the sexual stages of the parasite, the gametocytes, when it bites a malaria-infected person to take a blood meal. The gametocytes undergo further development in the insect for a period of 6–12 days, after which they are capable of infecting a human, again through the bite of the mosquito.

The intensity of malaria transmission in an area is the rate at which people are inoculated with malaria parasites by mosquitoes. It is usually expressed as the annual entomological inoculation rate (EIR), i.e. the average number of infectious bites by malaria-infected mosquitoes delivered to an individual human resident in the area in the period of one year. It is the EIR that determines, to a large extent, the epidemiology of malaria and the pattern of clinical disease in that locality. The high end of the malaria transmission range is found in a few parts of tropical Africa, where EIRs of 500–1000 can be reached *(1)*. At the low end of the range are EIRs of 0.01 or below, as found in the temperate climates of the Caucasus and Central Asia where malaria transmission is only barely sustained. Between these extremes are situations of unstable seasonal malaria such as in much of Asia and Latin America where EIRs lie below 10, and often around 1–2, and situations of stable but still seasonal malaria as in much of West Africa where the EIR is in the range 10–100.

The proportion of infected mosquitoes in a locality is itself related to the number of infected and infectious humans living there. Therefore, lowering of the infectivity of infected persons to the mosquito vector will contribute to lowering of malaria transmission, and eventually to reducing the prevalence of malaria and the incidence of disease in that locality. The relationship between the EIR and the prevalence of malaria is, however, complex and is affected by the nature of immunity to malaria, its acquisition and loss and to whether or not there is effective drug treatment. The hypothetical relationship represented in figure A4.1 assumes no drug treatment. In areas of low transmission, where EIRs are below 1 or 2, a reduction in the inoculation rates will result in an almost proportionate reduction in the prevalence (and incidence rate) of malaria. At EIRs in excess of 10, the reductions in transmission need to be increasingly large if they are to make a significant impact on malaria prevalence. In high-transmission settings where there is great redundancy in the infectious reservoir, the impact of reducing transmission on disease incidence is not at all obvious, and has been the subject of considerable debate. The experience with major interventions, such as the use of insecticide-treated nets, suggests, however, that effective transmission-reducing interventions will always be beneficial with respect to mortality *(2, 3)*.

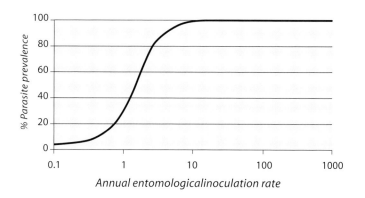

Figure A4.1   Relationship between inoculation rate and parasite prevalence (assumes that all infections are untreated)

A4.2   Effects of antimalarials on malaria transmission

Antimalarials can help bring about a reduction in malaria transmission by their effect on parasite infectivity. This can be a direct effect on the gametocytes, the infective stages found in human infections (gametocytocidal effect) or, when the drug is taken up in the blood meal of the mosquito, an effect on the parasite's development in the insect (sporonticidal effect) (Table A4.1; Figure A4.2). Chloroquine acts against young gametocytes but has no suppressive effects on mature infective forms *(4)*. Chloroquine has even been shown to be capable of enhancing the infectivity of gametocytes to the mosquito *(5)*. In contrast, sulfadoxine-pyrimethamine increases gametocyte carriage but, provided there is no resistance, reduces the infectivity of gametocytes to mosquitoes *(5–7)*. Artemisinins are the most potent gametocytocidal drugs among those currently being used to treat an asexual blood infection *(8–11)*. They destroy immature gametocytes, preventing new infective gametocytes from entering the circulation, but their effects on mature gametocytes are less and so they will not affect the infectivity of those already present in the circulation at the time a patient presents for treatment *(11)*.

Table A4.1 **Effects of some commonly used antimalarials on the infectivity of *P. falciparum* to the mosquito**

| Drug | Effect of treatment | | | |
| | Gametocytocidal | | Sporonticidal | Overall effect on suppressing infectivity[a] |
	Viability of young sequestered gametocytes	Viability of mature circulating gametocytes	Infectivity of gametocytes to mosquitoes	
Chloroquine	Reduces	No effect (4)	Enhances (5)	+
Sulfadoxine-pyrimethamine	No effect	Increases (5–7)	Suppresses (5–7)	+/–
Artemisinin derivatives	Reduces greatly (8–11)	Little effect (11)	Unknown	+++
Primaquine	Unknown	Reduces greatly (11)	Unknown	+++
Quinine (4)	No effect	No effect	No effect	None

[a] +/– no overall effect; + moderate effect; ++ high effect; +++ very high effect

Primaquine, an 8-aminoquinoline antimalarial that has been widely used as a hypnozoiticidal drug, is the only antimalarial medicine that had been deployed in the treatment of *P. falciparum* infections specifically for its effects on infectivity. It acts on mature infective gametocytes in the circulation and accelerates gametocyte clearance (11), as opposed to artemisinins which mainly inhibit gametocyte development.

A4.3 The use of antimalarials to reduce infectivity

A4.3.1 Choice of drugs

Artemisinin derivatives, as indicated earlier, have specific and significant activity against gametocytes (Table A3.1). Effective treatment of a malaria blood infection with any antimalarial will, nevertheless, remove the source of new gametocytes by eliminating the asexual blood stages from which gametocytes derive. The faster the clearance of asexual blood parasites by a drug, the greater will be its impact on infectivity. In *P. vivax, P. malariae* and *P. ovale* infections, in which gametocytes have a short developmental period and are short-lived, effective treatment of the asexual blood infection alone (without the addition of gametocytocidal drugs) will be sufficient to abolish further infectivity to mosquitoes. *P. falciparum* is different because its gametocytes take longer to develop – about 12 days to mature from a young parasite (merozoite) – and the mature gametocytes may remain infective in the peripheral circulation for up to several weeks after the patient has

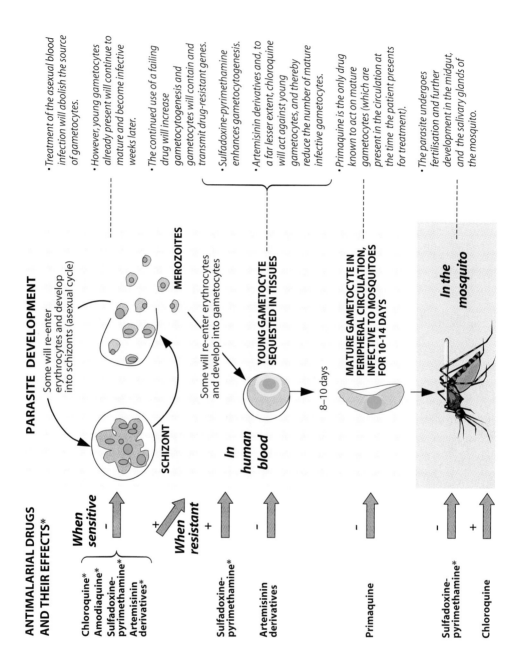

* When parasites are sensitive to the drug unless otherwise stated. Positive and negative arrows indicate the effect of the drug, enhancement (+) and suppression (-) respectively, on the parasite stage or its development.

Figure A4.2 Transmission of *Plasmodium falciparum* and the effects of antimalarials

been successfully treated for the asexual blood infection. In order to terminate infectivity of *P. falciparum*, the infection needs to be treated with drugs that have specific activity against gametocytes, i.e. either ACTs that destroy immature gametocytes, or by the addition of primaquine to the treatment regime to eradicate mature gametocytes. It is not known whether the use of primaquine with ACTs would result in a further suppression of infectivity, although it appears possible in principle, given that the two drugs act on different developmental stages of gametocytes.

A4.3.2 The effect on transmission of using transmission-blocking medicines

Situations of low to moderate transmission

The most direct consequences of lowering the infectivity of patients by the use of drugs are to be seen in areas of low transmission, where symptomatic patients constitute the majority of the infectious reservoir. Here, a strategy to shorten the period of infectivity of patients, if it could be achieved on a wide scale, would have a significant impact on the parasite reservoir of infection and, therefore, on malaria transmission. A reduction in transmission would, in these situations, result in an almost proportionate reduction in the prevalence of infection and incidence of disease.

In areas of low to moderate transmission, therefore, the provision of prompt and effective treatment to malaria patients is important both as a means of achieving the public health goal of reducing transmission, and attaining the therapeutic goal of reducing morbidity. Also important in these situations is the use of specific gametocytocidal drugs. There are anecdotal accounts from areas of low transmission with inadequate health services that offer little access to treatment, of patients presenting with extremely high parasite prevalence rates (>70%), approaching those found in areas of intense transmission (Figure A4.1). When treatment centres were established in such areas and early and effective malaria treatment was provided to patients, parasite prevalence and disease incidence rates decreased dramatically. One well-documented example is from the north-western border of Thailand where high incidence rates of *P. falciparum* prevailed in the face of increasing resistance to mefloquine, the antimalarial in use at the time. There, the deployment of artesunate in combination with mefloquine led to a significant decline in the incidence of the disease *(12)*.

Situations of intense transmission

In high-transmission settings, infected but asymptomatic persons constitute an important part of the infectious reservoir. Even though treated cases (mainly children) have higher densities of gametocytes, and effectiveness of transmission is positively related to gametocyte density, a treatment strategy to reduce infectivity of patients whose contribution to the reservoir of infection is only partial is not likely to have a major impact on transmission. This, together with the fact that a much greater reduction in transmission rates needs to be achieved in order to reduce parasite prevalence (and incidence of disease), makes the case for introducing an infectivity-suppressing component to the drug treatment of patients less compelling as a strategy for reducing the incidence of disease. However, the potentially important role of medication in reducing transmission must not be overlooked even in these situations. As intensified malaria control efforts deploying highly effective interventions, such as use of insecticide-treated mosquito nets and indoor residual spraying with insecticides, get under way, malaria inoculation rates could fall considerably *(13)*. Transmission-reducing drug regimes will then have a greater role to play, and will complement other methods to achieve an impact on mortality and the incidence of malaria.

The use of antimalarial drugs to reduce infectivity:

- **is essential in low-transmission settings,**
- **will be beneficial in high-transmission settings if used in conjunction with other effective transmission-blocking interventions.**

A4.4 Dynamics of drug pressure and transmission of drug-resistant genes

A4.4.1 The continued use of a failing drug will confer a selective transmission advantage to resistant parasites

It has been shown that when resistance to a drug is prevalent in a locality, the continued use of that drug will confer a selective advantage to parasites carrying resistance genes, and will lead to higher rates of transmission of drug-resistant parasites. This will result in the rapid spread of the drug resistance through two mechanisms. First the use of the drug leads to higher numbers of circulating gametocytes in the resistant infections than in the sensitive ones *(5, 6, 9, 10, 14, 15)*. The failing drug may reduce asexual para-sitaemias initially to an extent that they may be undetectable even by PCR, but it induces the production of detectable numbers of gametocytes carrying the resistant genes. Resistance is associated with recrudescence. The subsequent recrudescence is associated with higher rates of gametocyte carriage than the primary infection. The recrudescence with resistance parasites is also more likely to fail treatment and recrudesce again than the primary infection. Thus cumulatively the resistant infection generates more gametocytes than an infection with sensitive parasites. Secondly, gametocytes carrying resistant genes have been shown to be more infectious to mosquitoes. They produce higher densities of parasites (oocysts) in the mosquitoes, and infect a higher proportion of mosquitoes than those carrying sensitive genes *(6, 7, 11)*. Molecular studies on the transmission of two *P. falciparum* genes linked to chloroquine resistance, *pfcrt* and *pfmdr*, showed that gametocytes carrying the former produced more oocysts and were also more infectious to mosquitoes than gametocytes of the sensitive genotype *(15)*.

A4.4.2   Reversal of transmission advantage by artemisinins

The use of drugs in combination, specifically with artemisinin derivatives, will remove the survival advantage conferred on parasites resistant to a particular drug by the use of that drug as monotherapy *(10, 15, 16)*. This is because artemisinins are very effective in clearing blood parasites and also in reducing gametocyte prevalence and density *(10)*, and therefore infectivity. But high cure rates are needed to prevent recrudescence with its greater carriage, and so it is inadvisable to combine an artemisinin derivative with a failing partner drug. Artemisinins have a short *in vivo* half-life so that their gametocytocidal activity will soon cease, leaving the parasites exposed to the failing partner drug, which has a longer *in vivo* half-life. There is a high failure rate and transmission of resistance parasites is not prevented *(9, 10, 15)*. The clear advantage of using artemisinins in combination with an effective partners drug is that it will delay the selection and spread of drug-resistant genes *(10–12, 15, 16)*.

The implications are as follows.

- Once drug resistance has emerged in a locality, the continued use of the failing drug will result in:
  - the rapid spread of drug resistance in the area because the use of the drug confers a transmission advantage to resistant parasites;
  - the prevalence of infections in which only gametocytes may be present in the peripheral circulation; the continued use of the drug can lead to low-grade asexual parasitaemias with a high rate of differentiation to gametocytes; such infections must be considered as active drug-resistant infections and be treated with an effective second-line medicine.
- Early treatment of malaria patients with an effective antimalarial has the greatest chance of limiting the spread of drug-resistant parasites.
- The use of an artemisinin derivative with an effective partner drug will delay the selection and spread of drug resistance.

A4.5 The role of transmission-blocking interventions and antimalarials in curtailing the spread of drug resistance

A4.5.1 Transmission control

A reduction in transmission will curtail the spread of parasites of both sensitive and resistant strains. However, there is evidence to suggest that, in the absence of drug pressure, resistant parasites are at a survival disadvantage compared to sensitive strains, i.e. in the absence of selection by the drug to which they are resistant, drug-resistant parasites tend to be intrinsically less able to be transmitted than are drug-sensitive parasites (17, 18). These more stringent transmission conditions will, therefore, tend to selectively eliminate drug-resistant parasites (19). This expectation is supported by observations in Zimbabwe, where house spraying with insecticides to reduce malaria transmission was associated with reductions in the amount of drug resistance in the malaria parasites (20). Likewise, in low-transmission settings in India and Sri Lanka, the replacement of the failing chloroquine with an effective antimalarial, in combination with intense entomological transmission control, led to significant reductions, and in some instances even elimination, of chloroquine-resistant *P. falciparum*. In western Thailand where, in the 1990s, increasing levels of mefloquine resistance were associated with rising malaria incidence, the deployment of combination therapy for malaria treatment with mefloquine and artesunate was associated with an increased *in vitro* suscepti-bility of *P. falciparum* to mefloquine (12).

A4.5.2 Antimalarials

In contrast to transmission control methods, such as residual insecticide spraying and the use of insecticide-treated nets – which are constantly in effect against the entire parasite population through the killing of the vector mosquito and the prevention of biting – treatment with antimalarials affects only the parasites in an infected person at the time of treatment. In high-transmission situations, this is a relatively rare event because the proportion of persons who are ill among those who are infected is quite small, and applies only to a small fraction of the parasite population. Therefore, the impact of drug treatment as a means of curtailing the spread of resistant parasites may be small in comparison to that of vector control methods.

The implications are as follows:

- **The implementation of transmission control through vector control methods will help reduce the spread of drug resistance.**
- **The use of infectivity-suppressing medicines will be synergistic with mosquito control methods.**

A4.6 Conclusion

In situations of low malaria transmission, antimalarials have been and are being used for the specific purpose of reducing infectivity to mosquitoes – a notable example being the use of primaquine in the treatment of *P. falciparum* malaria. In areas of intense transmission, however, suppression of parasite infectivity has previously not been regarded as a significant goal of treatment. Now, the situation has changed. Artemisinin derivatives (which are gametocytocidal as well as destroying asexual stages of the parasite) are being widely deployed for the treatment of malarial disease, including in areas of intense transmission. This will allow the impact of anti-infective drugs on the reservoir of infection and transmission rates to be evaluated across the entire range of transmission intensities.

Reducing transmission is fundamental to the curtailment of drug resistance, and antimalarials can help achieve this, at least in some situations. This has implications for malaria treatment policy and also for drug development. The ability to suppress parasite infectivity should be included in the product profile of compounds that are being evaluated as potential new antimalarials.

A4.7 References

1. Hay SI et al. Annual *Plasmodium falciparum* entomological inoculation rates (EIR) across Africa: literature survey, Internet access and review. *Transactions of the Royal Society of Tropical Medicine and Hygiene*, 2000, 94:113–127.

2. Lengeler C, Smith TA, Armstrong-Schellenberg J. Focus on the effect of bed nets on malaria morbidity and mortality. *Parasitology Today*, 1997, 13:123–124.

3. Molineaux L. Malaria and mortality: some epidemiological considerations. *Annals of Tropical Medicine and Parasitology*, 1997, 91:811–825.

4. Bruce-Chwatt L. *Chemotherapy of malaria*, 2nd ed. Geneva, World Health Organization, 1981:261.

5. Hogh B et al. The differing impact of chloroquine and pyrimethamine/sulfadoxine upon the infectivity of malaria species to the mosquito vector. *American Jour* of *Tropical Medicine and Hygiene*, 1998, 58:176–182.

6. Robert V et al. Gametocytemia and infectivity to mosquitoes of patients with uncomplicated, *Plasmodium falciparum* malaria attacks treated with chloroquine or sulfadoxine plus pyrimethamine. *American Journal of Tropical Medicine and Hygiene*, 2000, 62:210–216.

7. von Seidlein L et al. Risk factors for gametocyte carriage in Gambian children. *American Journal of Tropical Medicine and Hygiene*, 2001, 65:523–527.

8. von Seidlein L et al. A randomized controlled trial of artemether/benflumetol, a new antimalarial, and pyrimethamine/sulfadoxine in the treatment of uncomplicated falciparum malaria in African children. *American Journal of Tropical Medicine and Hygiene*, 1998, 58:638–644.

9. Targett G et al. Artesunate reduces but does not prevent post-treatment transmission of *Plasmodium falciparum* to *Anopheles gambiae*. *Journal of Infectious Diseases*, 2001, 183:1254–1259.

10. Drakeley CJ et al. Addition of artesunate to chloroquine for treatment of *Plasmodium falciparum* malaria in Gambian children causes a significant but short-lived reduction in infectiousness for mosquitoes. *Tropical Medicine and International Health*, 2004, 9:53–61.

11. Pukrittayakamee S et al. Activities of artesunate and primaquine against asexual- and sexual-stage parasites in falciparum malaria. *Antimicrobial Agents and Chemotherapy*, 2004, 48:1329–1334.

12. Nosten F et al. Effects of artesunate-mefloquine combination on incidence of *Plasmodium falciparum* malaria and mefloquine resistance in western Thailand: a prospective study. *Lancet*, 2000, 356:297–302.

13. Killeem G et al. The potential impact of integrated malaria transmission control on entomologic inoculation rate in highly endemic areas. *American Journal of Tropical Medicine and Hygiene*, 2000, 62:545–551.

14. Handunnetti SM et al. Features of recrudescent chloroquine-resistant *Plasmodium falciparum* infections confer a survival advantage on parasites, and have implications for disease control. *Transactions of the Royal Society of Tropical Medicine and Hygiene*, 1996, 90:563–567.

15. Hallett RL et al. Combination therapy counteracts the enhanced transmission of drug-resistant malaria parasites to mosquitoes. *Antimicrobial Agents and Chemotherapy*, 2004, 48:3940–3943.

16. White NJ, Olliaro PL. Strategies for the prevention of antimalarial drug resistance: rationale for combination chemotherapy for malaria. *Parasitology Today*, 1996, 12:399–401.

17. De Roode JC et al. Competitive release of drug resistance following drug treatment of mixed *Plasmodium chabaudi* infections. *Malaria Journal*, 2004, 3:33–42.

18. De Roode JC et al. Host heterogeneity is a determinant of competitive exclusion or coexistence in genetically diverse malaria infections. *Proceedings of the Royal Society of London B, Biological Sciences*, 2004, 271:1073–1080.

19. Molyneux DH et al. Transmission control and drug resistance in malaria: a crucial interaction. *Parasitology Today*, 1999, 15:238–240.

20. Mharakurwa S et al. Association of house spraying with suppressed levels of drug resistance in Zimbabwe. *Malaria Journal*, 2004, 3:35.

Annex 5. Malaria diagnosis

ANNEX 5

MALARIA DIAGNOSIS

A5.1 Symptom-based (clinical) diagnosis

The signs and symptoms of malaria, such as fever, chills, headache and anorexia, are non-specific and are common to many diseases and conditions. Malaria is a common cause of fever and illness in endemic areas (1, 2), but it is not possible to apply any one set of clinical criteria to the diagnosis of all types of malaria in all patient populations. The appropriateness of particular clinical diagnostic criteria varies from area to area according to the intensity of transmission, the species of malaria parasite, other prevailing causes of fever, and the health service infrastructure (3). One of the factors leading to a change in the clinical epidemiology of malaria in some areas is the prevalence of HIV/AIDS. This disease can increase the risk of acquiring malaria or the progression to severe malaria, depending on malaria transmission in the area and the age of the patient. The prevalence of HIV/AIDS can also lead to an increase in the incidence of febrile disease that is not malaria, and can therefore cause further difficulties in the symptom-based diagnosis of malaria (4).

Two different studies in The Gambia have shown that a sensitivity of 70–88% and a specificity of 63–82% for malaria diagnosis could be achieved using a weighting and scoring system for clinical signs and symptoms. These methods may be too complicated to implement and supervise under operational conditions in the field, and many of the key symptoms and signs of malaria in one area may not be applicable elsewhere. For instance, reduced feeding in a child is more likely to indicate malaria in The Gambia than in Ethiopia (5, 6).

Fever alone is as effective a criterion for diagnosis as clinical algorithms; a review of 10 studies indicated that use of the more restrictive criteria of clinical algorithms resulted in only trivial savings in drug costs compared with use of a fever-based diagnosis, even in areas of low malaria prevalence. In areas of high prevalence it greatly increases the probability of missing malaria infections (7).

A5.2 Light microscopy

In addition to providing a diagnosis with a high degree of sensitivity and specificity when performed well, microscopy allows quantification of malaria parasites and identification of the infecting species. It is inexpensive, the cost varying from US$ 0.40–0.70 per slide and is considered to be the "gold standard" against which the sensitivity and specificity of other methods must be assessed. A skilled microscopist is able to detect asexual parasites at densities of fewer than 10 per μl of blood but under typical field conditions the limit of sensitivity is approximately 100 parasites per μl *(8)*. Light microscopy has important advantages:

- low direct costs if the infrastructure to maintain the service is available,
- high sensitivity if the quality of microscopy is high,
- differentiation between plasmodia species,
- determination of parasite densities,
- can be used to diagnose many other conditions.

It can be difficult to maintain good quality of microscopy, for various reasons: the need for adequate training and supervision of laboratory staff; the need to rely on electricity at night time; delays in providing results to patients; and the need for maintaining quality assurance and control of laboratory services.

Numerous attempts have been made to improve malaria microscopy, but none has proven superior to the classical method of Giemsa-staining and oil-immersion microscopy for performance in typical health-care settings *(9)*.

A5.3   Rapid diagnostic tests

Rapid diagnostic tests (RDTs) are immunochromatographic tests that detect parasite-specific antigens in a finger-prick blood sample. Some tests detect only one species (*Plasmodium falciparum*), others detect one or more of the other three species of human malaria parasites (*P. vivax*, *P. malariae* and *P. ovale*) *(10–12)*. RDTs are available commercially in different formats, as dipsticks, cassettes or cards. Cassettes and cards are easier to use in difficult conditions outside health facilities.

RDTs are simple to perform and interpret, and do not require electricity or special equipment. WHO recommends that such tests should have a sensitivity of > 95% in detecting plasmodia at densities of more than 100 parasites per μl of blood. Programme and project managers should make their own choice among the many products available, using the criteria recommended by WHO (www.wpro. who.int/rdt) as there is as yet no international mechanism for pre-qualification of RDTs.

Current tests are based on the detection of histidine-rich protein 2 (HRP2), which is specific for *P. falciparum*, pan-specific or species-specific parasite lactate dehydrogenase (pLDH), or other pan-specific antigens such as aldolase. These antigens have different characteristics, which may affect suitability for use in different situations, and this should be taken into account when developing RDT policy. These tests have many potential advantages, including:

- the ability to provide rapid results,
- fewer requirements for training and skilled personnel (a general health worker can be trained in one day),
- reinforcement of patient confidence in the diagnosis and in the health service in general.

There are also potential disadvantages, including:

- the likelihood of misinterpreting a positive result as indicating malaria in patients with parasitaemia incidental to another illness, in particular when host immunity is high; the inability in the case of some RDTs, to distinguish new infections from a recently and effectively treated infection; this is due to the persistence of certain target antigens (e.g. HRP2) in the blood for 1–3 weeks after effective treatment. The persistence of PfHRP2 in blood for at least one week after treatment can be used in the diagnosis of severe malaria in low transmission areas where artemisinin derivatives are widely available. Patients may have cleared peripheral parasitaemia because of inadequate self treatment, but the PfHRP2 test will be strongly positive.
- unpredictable sensitivity in the field *(13–20),* mainly because test performance is greatly affected by adverse environmental conditions such as high temperature and humidity.

Published sensitivities of RDTs for *P. falciparum* range from comparable to those of good field microscopy (>90% at 100–500 parasites/µl of blood) to very poor (40–50%) for some widely used products. Sensitivities are generally lower for other species. The reasons for poor sensitivity are not clear. They may include: poor test manufacture, damage due to exposure to high temperature or humidity, incorrect handling by end-users, possible geographical variation in the test antigen, and poor comparative microscopy *(12)*. Several studies have shown that health workers, volunteers and private sector providers can, with some support and follow-up, learn to use RDTs correctly with relative ease.

The use of a confirmatory diagnosis with either microscopy or RDTs is expected to reduce the overuse of antimalarials by ensuring that treatment is targeted on patients with confirmed malaria infections as opposed to treating all patients with fever. There is, however, little documented evidence that this is so. The main problem is that providers of care, although they may be willing to perform diagnostic tests, do not always comply with the results, especially when they are negative. Being aware that delay in providing effective treatment can be fatal for a malaria patient, they are often reluctant to withhold treatment on the basis of a negative result. WHO is currently supporting operational research projects designed to address these issues.

A5.4 Immunodiagnosis and PCR-based molecular detection methods

Detection of antibodies to parasites, which may be useful for epidemiological studies, is neither sensitive, specific, nor rapid enough to be of use in the management of patients suspected of having malaria *(21)*.

Techniques to detect parasite DNA based on the polymerase chain reaction (PCR) are highly sensitive and very useful for detecting mixed infections, in particular at low parasite densities. They are also useful for studies on drug resistance and other specialized epidemiological investigations *(22)*, but are not generally available in malaria endemic areas.

What are the effects of treatment based on clinical diagnosis compared with treatment based on diagnosis with the use of malaria microscopy or RDTs?[a]

Interventions: use of RDTs or microscopy for diagnosis

Summary of RCTs: despite the existence of a number of studies on the sensitivity and specificity of various methods for diagnosing malaria, there are no RCTs on the impact of a confirmatory diagnosis as an intervention.

Expert comment: treatment of all people with fever leads to overuse of antimalarials in most settings. With the introduction of more expensive antimalarials, there is a need to target treatment more effectively on people with malaria infections by using confirmatory testing. This will have the additional benefits of improving patient care and providing better epidemiological surveillance data. However, in young children in areas of intense transmission, it is believed that the risk associated with relying on a parasitological diagnosis (death owing to a false negative result) may outweigh the benefits.

Recommendation: except for children in areas of intense transmission, confirmatory (parasitological) testing should be introduced and used to supplement clinical criteria in diagnosis.

Controlled trials and operational research in various settings are urgently needed.

[a] See also references (7) and (23).

A5.5   References

1. Marsh K et al. Clinical algorithm for malaria in Africa. *Lancet*, 1996, 347:1327–1329.

2. Redd SC et al. Clinical algorithm for treatment of *Plasmodium falciparum* in children. *Lancet*, 347:223–227.

3. *WHO Expert Committee on Malaria. Twentieth report.* Geneva, World Health Organization, 2000 (WHO Technical Report Series, No. 892).

4. Nwanyanwu OC et al. Malaria and human immunodeficiency virus infection among male employees of a sugar estate in Malawi. *Transactions of the Royal Society of Tropical Medicine and Hygiene*, 1997, 91:567–569.

5. Bojang KA, Obaro S, Morison LA. A prospective evaluation of a clinical algorithm for the diagnosis of malaria in Gambian children. *Tropical Medicine and International Health*, 2000, 5:231–236.

6. Olaleye BO et al. Clinical predictors of malaria in Gambian children with fever or a history of fever. *Transactions of the Royal Society of Tropical Medicine and Hygiene*, 1998, 92:300–304.

7. Chandramohan D, Jaffar S, Greenwood B. Use of clinical algorithms for diagnosing malaria. *Tropical Medicine and International Health*, 2002, 7, 45–52.

8. World Health Organization. Malaria diagnosis. Memorandum from a WHO meeting. *Bulletin of the World Health Organization*, 1988, 66:575.

9. Kawamoto F, Billingsley PF. Rapid diagnosis of malaria by fluorescence microscopy. *Parasitology Today*, 1992, 8:69–71.

10. *Malaria diagnosis: new perspectives.* Geneva, World Health Organization, 2000 (document WHO/CDS/RBM/2000.14).

11. *Malaria rapid diagnosis: making it work.* Geneva, World Health Organization, 2003 (document RS/2003/GE/05(PHL)).

12. *The use of rapid diagnostic tests.* Geneva, Roll Back Malaria, WHO Regional Office for the Western Pacific and UNDP/World Bank/WHO/UNICEF Special Programme for Research and Training in Tropical Diseases, 2004.

13. Gaye O et al. Diagnosis of *Plasmodium falciparum* malaria using ParaSight F, ICT malaria PF and malaria IgG CELISA assays. *Parasite*, 1998, 5: 189–192.

14. Ricci L et al. Evaluation of OptiMAL Assay test to detect imported malaria in Italy. *New Microbiology*, 2000, 23: 391–398.

15. Iqbal J et al. Diagnosis of imported malaria by *Plasmodium* lactate dehydrogenase (pLDH) and histidine-rich protein 2 (PfHRP-2)-based immunocapture assays. *American Journal of Tropical Medicine and Hygiene*, 2001, 64:20–23.

16. Rubio JM et al. Limited level of accuracy provided by available rapid diagnosis tests for malaria enhances the need for PCR-based reference laboratories. *Journal of Clinical Microbiology*, 39: 2736–2737.

17. Coleman R et al. Field evaluation of the ICT Malaria Pf/Pv immunochromatographic test for the detection of asymptomatic malaria in a *Plasmodium falciparum/vivax* endemic area in Thailand. *American Journal of Tropical Medicine and Hygiene*, 2002, 66:379–383.

18. Craig MH et al. Field and laboratory comparative evaluation of ten rapid malaria diagnostic tests. *Transactions of the Royal Society of Tropical Medicine and Hygiene*, 2002, 96:258–265.

19. Huong NM et al. Comparison of three antigen detection methods for diagnosis and therapeutic monitoring of malaria: a field study from southern Vietnam. *Tropical Medicine and International Health*, 7:304–308.

20. Mason DP et al. A comparison of two rapid field immunochromatographic tests to expert microscopy in the diagnosis of malaria. *Acta Tropica*, 2002, 82: 51–59.

21. Voller A. The immunodiagnosis of malaria. In: Wernsdorfer WH, McGregor I. *Malaria*, Vol.1. Edinburgh, Churchill Livingstone, 1988:815–827.

22. Bates I, Iboro J, Barnish G. Challenges in monitoring the impact of interventions against malaria using diagnostics. In: *Reducing malaria's burden. Evidence of effectiveness for decision-makers*. Washington DC, Global Health Council, 2003:33–39 (Global Health Council Technical Report).

23. *Role of parasitological diagnosis in malaria case management in areas of high transmission. Summary of the outcomes of a WHO Technical Consultation held in Geneva, 25–26 October 2004.* Geneva, World Health Organization (in preparation).

Annex 6.   Resistance to antimalarials

ANNEX 6

RESISTANCE TO ANTIMALARIALS

A6.1 Introduction

There are currently no bedside tests for determining the susceptibility of the malaria parasite to antimalarials. Monitoring is therefore needed to determine geographical trends in susceptibility and the emergence and spread of drug resistance. The information obtained will help guide treatment choices and predictions about future resistance patterns.

The greatest problem with drug resistance occur with *P. falciparum*. Resistance of *P. falciparum* is of particular concern because of the enormous burden of disease caused by this species, its lethal potential, the propensity for epidemics, and the cost of candidate replacement drugs for areas with established drug resistance. Chloroquine resistance does occur in *P. vivax,* especially in western Oceania, but there are very few reports of resistance in *P. malariae* or *P. ovale* (although there have also been very few studies).

This annex defines resistance, examines how it arises and spreads, summarizes its current global distribution and describes ways in which it can be monitored.

A6.2 Definition

Antimalarial drug resistance is defined as the ability of a parasite strain to survive and/or multiply despite the proper administration and absorption of an antimalarial drug in the dose normally recommended. Drug resistance to an antimalarial compound results in a right shift in the concentration–effect (dose–response) relationship (Figure A6.1). As the pharmacokinetic properties of antimalarials vary widely in different individuals, the definition of resistance should probably also include a "normal" plasma concentration profile for the active drug concerned or, in the case of a prodrug (a drug that is not active in the ingested form and requires chemical conversion through metabolic processes to become pharmacologically active), a "normal" profile of the biologically active metabolite. Antimalarial drug resistance is not necessarily the same as malaria "treatment failure", which is a failure to clear malarial parasitaemia and/or resolve clinical symptoms despite the administration of an antimalarial. So while drug resistance may lead to treatment failure, not all treatment failures are caused by drug resistance. Treatment failure can also be the result of incorrect dosing, problems of treatment adherence (compliance), poor drug quality, interactions with other drugs, compromised drug absorption, or misdiagnosis of the patient. Apart from leading to inappropriate case management, all these factors may also accelerate the spread of true drug resistance by exposure of the parasites to inadequate drug levels.

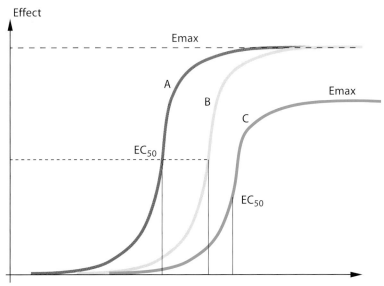

Figure A6.1 **Resistance is a rightward shift in the concentration–effect relationship for a particular parasite population. This may be a parallel shift (B) from the "normal" profile (A) or, in some circumstances, the slope changes, and/or the maximum achievable effect is reduced (C). The effect is parasite killing**

A6.3 The emergence and spread of antimalarial resistance

The development of resistance can be considered in two parts: the initial genetic event, which produces the resistant mutant; and the subsequent selection process in which the survival advantage in the presence of the drug leads to preferential transmission of resistant mutants and thus the spread of resistance. In the absence of the antimalarial, resistant mutants may have a survival disadvantage. This "fitness cost" of the resistance mechanism may result in a decline in the prevalence of resistance once drug pressure is removed.

Resistance to one drug may select for resistance to another where the mechanisms of resistance are similar (cross-resistance). There are many parallels with antibiotic resistance, in particular resistance to antituberculosis drugs where, as for malaria, transferable resistance genes are not involved in the emergence of resistance *(1–3)*. In experimental models, drug-resistant mutations can be selected without mosquito passage (i.e. without meiotic recombination) by exposure of large numbers of malaria parasites (either *in vitro*, in animals, or as was done in the past, in volunteers) to subtherapeutic drug concentrations *(4)*.

Various factors determine the propensity for antimalarial drug resistance to develop *(5)*:

- the intrinsic frequency with which the genetic changes occur,
- the degree of resistance (the shift in the concentration-effect relationship, (Figure A6.1) conferred by the genetic change,
- the fitness cost of the resistance mechanism,
- the proportion of all transmissible infections that are exposed to the drug (the selection pressure),
- the number of parasites exposed to the drug,
- the concentrations of drug to which these parasites are exposed ,
- the pharmacokinetic and pharmacodynamic properties of the antimalarial,
- individual (dosing, duration, adherence) and community (quality, availability, distribution) patterns of drug use,
- the immunity profile of the community and the individual,
- the simultaneous presence of other antimalarials or substances in the blood to which the parasite is not resistant.

The emergence of resistance can be thought of in terms of the product of the probabilities of *de novo* emergence (a rare event) and subsequent spread. Resistant parasites, if present, will be selected when parasites are exposed to "selective" (subtherapeutic) drug concentrations. "Selective" in this context means a concentration of drug that will eradicate the sensitive parasites but still allow growth of the resistant parasite population such that it eventually transmits to another person. Because *de novo* resistance arises randomly among malaria parasites, non-immune patients infected with large numbers of parasites who receive inadequate treatment (either because of poor drug quality, poor adherence, vomiting of an oral treatment, etc.) are a potent source of *de novo* resistance. This emphasizes the importance of correct prescribing, and good adherence to prescribed drug regimens, and also provision of treatment regimens that are still highly effective in hyperparasitaemic patients. The principle specific immune response that controls the primary symptomatic infection in falciparum malaria is directed by the variant surface antigen (PfEMP1). The parasite population evades this immune response by switching its surface antigen in a specific sequence of changes. The probability of selecting a resistant parasite from the primary infection is the product of the switch rate and the rate of formation of viable resistant parasites.

The subsequent spread of resistant mutant malaria parasites is facilitated by the widespread use of drugs with long elimination phases. These provide a "selective filter", allowing infection by the resistant parasites while the residual antimalarial activity prevents infection by sensitive parasites. Slowly eliminated drugs such as mefloquine (terminal elimination half-life ($T_{1/2}\beta$ 2–3 weeks) or chloroquine ($T_{1/2}\beta$ 1–2 months) persist in the blood and provide a selective filter for months after drug administration has ceased.

A6.3.1 Transmission intensity and the selection and spread of resistance

The recrudescence and subsequent transmission of an infection that has generated a *de novo* resistant malaria parasite is essential for resistance to be propagated *(5)*. Gametocytes carrying the resistance genes will not reach transmissible densities until the resistant biomass has expanded to numbers close to those producing illness (>10^7 parasites) *(6)*. Thus to prevent resistance spreading from an infection that has generated *de novo* resistance, gametocyte production from the recrudescent resistant infection must be prevented. There has been debate as to whether resistance arises more rapidly in low- or high-transmission settings *(7, 8)*, but aside from theoretical calculations, epidemiological studies clearly implicate low-transmission settings as the source of drug resistance. Chloroquine resistance and high-level sulfadoxine-pyrimethamine resistance in *P. falciparum* both originated in South-East Asia and subsequently spread to Africa *(9)*.

In low-transmission areas, the majority of malaria infections are symptomatic and selection therefore takes place in the context of treatment. Relatively large numbers of parasites in an individual usually encounter antimalarials at concentrations that are maximally effective. But in a variable proportion of patients, for the reasons mentioned earlier, blood concentrations are low and may select for resistance.

In high-transmission areas, the majority of infections are asymptomatic and infections are acquired repeatedly throughout life. Symptomatic and sometimes fatal malaria occurs in the first years of life, but thereafter it is increasingly likely to be asymptomatic. This reflects a state of imperfect immunity (premunition), where the infection is controlled, usually at levels below those causing symptoms. The rate at which premunition is acquired depends on the intensity of transmission. In the context of intense malaria transmission, people still receive antimalarial treatments throughout their lives (often inappropriately for other febrile infections), but these "treatments" are largely unrelated to the peaks of parasitaemia, thereby reducing the probability of selection for resistance.

Immunity considerably reduces the emergence of resistance (9). Host defence contributes a major antiparasitic effect, and any spontaneously generated drug-resistant mutant malaria parasite must contend not only with the concentrations of antimalarial present, but also with host immunity. This kills parasites regardless of their antimalarial resistance, and reduces the probability of parasite survival (independently of drugs) at all stages of the transmission cycle. For the blood stage infection, immunity acts in a similar way to anti-malarials both to eliminate the rare *de novo* resistant mutants and stop them being transmitted (i.e. like a combination therapy), and also to improve cure rates with failing drugs (i.e. drugs falling to resistance) thereby reducing the relative transmission advantage of resistant parasites. Even if a resistant mutant does survive the initial drug treatment and multiplies, the chance that this will result in sufficient gametocytes for transmission is reduced as a result of asexual stage immunity (which reduces the multiplication rate and lowers the density at which the infection is controlled) and transmission-blocking immunity. Furthermore, other parasite genotypes are likely to be present, competing with the resistant parasites for red cells, and increasing the possibility of outbreeding of multigenic resistance mechanisms or competition in the feeding anopheline mosquito (10).

A6.3.2 Antimalarial pharmacodynamics and the selection of resistance

The genetic events that confer antimalarial drug resistance (while retaining parasite viability) are spontaneous and rare. They are thought to be independent of the drug. The resistance mechanisms that have been described are mutations in genes or changes in the copy number of genes relating to the drug's target or pumps that affect intraparasitic concentrations of the drug. A single genetic event may be all that is required, or multiple unlinked events may be necessary (epistasis). *P. falciparum* parasites from South-East Asia seem constitutionally to have an increased propensity to develop drug resistance.

Aminoquinolines

Chloroquine resistance in *P. falciparum* may be multigenic and is initially conferred by mutations in a gene that encodes a transporter (PfCRT). PfCRT may be an anion channel pumping chloroquine out from the food vacuole. The initial mutation, which confers a moderate level of chloroquine resistance, is replacement of a lysine with threonine at codon 76. Positions 72 to 76 are critical for the binding of desethylamodiaquine (the biologically active metabolite of amodiaquine) and also verapamil (which may reverse chloroquine resistance *in vitro*). Eleven other PfCRT mutations have been described to date. These additional mutations may contribute to aminoquinoline resistance, although the precise mechanisms have not yet been determined. Amodiaquine resistance is linked to chloroquine resistance, but is not well characterized. In the presence of PfCRT mutations, point mutations in a second transporter (PfMDR1) modulate the level of *P. falciparum* resistance *in vitro*. Parasites that are highly resistant to chloroquine often have Lys76Thr and Ala220Ser in PfCRT, and Asn86Tyr in PfMDR. The role of PfMDR1 mutations in determining the therapeutic response following chloroquine treatment is still unclear. The cause of chloroquine resistance in *P. vivax* has not been found yet.

Mefloquine

Resistance to mefloquine and other structurally related aryl-amino-alcohols in *P. falciparum* results from amplifications (i.e. duplications not mutations) in *Pfmdr*, which encodes an energy-demanding *p*-glycoprotein pump. This explains approximately two-thirds of the variance in susceptibility. Interestingly, it appears that generally only the "wild type" (PfMDR Asn86) amplifies, so that in the transition from chloroquine resistance, back mutation from mutant to wild type precedes amplification. Gene duplication is particularly frequent in the *P. falciparum* genome. It is a much more common genetic event than mutation. The low background frequency of gene amplification suggests that it may well confer a fitness disadvantage in the absence of selective pressure.

The products of these various genetic events result in reduced intracellular concentrations of the antimalarial quinolines in the parasite (the relative importance of reduced uptake and increased efflux remains unresolved).

Antifolate antimalarials

For the antifolate antimalarials (pyrimethamine, and the biguanides cycloguanil and chlorcycloguanil – the active metabolites of proguanil and chlorproguanil, respectively) resistance in *P. falciparum* and *P. vivax* results from the sequential acquisition of mutations in the gene *(dhfr)* that encodes dihydrofolate reductase (DHFR). Each mutation confers a stepwise reduction in susceptibility. In *P. falciparum*, the initial mutation is almost invariably at position 108 (usually serine to asparagine), which confers only a ten-fold reduction in drug susceptibility, and does not affect therapeutic responses to sulfadoxine-pyrimethamine. This has little clinical relevance initially, but then mutations arise at positions 51 and 59, conferring increasing resistance to pyrimethamine containing medicines. Infections with triple mutants are relatively resistant but some therapeutic response is usually seen. The acquisition of a fourth and devastating mutation at position 164 (isoleucine to leucine) renders the available antifolates completely ineffective (11). Interestingly, mutations conferring moderate pyrimethamine resistance do not necessarily confer cycloguanil resistance, and vice versa. For example, mutations at positions 16 (alanine to valine) plus 108 (serine to threonine) confer high-level resistance to cycloguanil but not to pyrimethamine. In general, the biguanides are more active than pyrimethamine against the resistant mutants (and they are more effective clinically too), but they are ineffective against parasites with the DHFR mutation at position 164. P. vivax shares similar antifolate resistance mechanisms through serial acquisition of mutations in PvDHFR. The sequence of acquisition associated with increasing resistance is usually mutation at position 117 or 58, followed by mutation at positions 57, 61 and then 13.

Sulfonamide and sulfone

The marked synergy with sulfonamides and sulfones is very important for the antimalarial activity of sulfa-pyrimethamine or sulfone-biguanide combinations. In P. falciparum, sulfonamide and sulfone resistance also develops by progressive acquisition of mutations in the gene encoding the target enzyme PfDHPS (which is a bifunctional protein with the enzyme PPPK). Specifically altered amino acid residues have been found at positions 436, 437, 540, 581 and 613 in the PfDHPS domain. The mutations at positions 581 and 631 do not occur in isolation, but always following an initial mutation (usually at position 437, alanine to glycine). Mutations in P. vivax DHPS (at positions 383 and 553) also appear to contribute to resistance.

Atovaquone-proguanil

Resistance to atovaquone results from point mutations in the gene (cytB), which encodes cytochrome b. In the atovaquone-proguanil combination, it is proguanil itself probably acting on the mitochondrial membrane rather than the dhfr-inhibiting proguanil metabolite cycloguanil that appears to be important in this combination. Whether and how resistance develops to the mitochondrial action of proguanil is not known.

Artemisinins

Although a target for the artemisinins has recently been identified (PfATPase6), preliminary studies have not so far associated polymorphisms in the gene encoding this enzyme with reduced susceptibility of malaria parasites. Amplification in PfMDR does reduce artemisinin susceptibility in vitro, but not to a degree that causes in vivo resistance. This has lead to erroneous claims that artemisinin resistance was being selected by widespread use of artemisinin derivatives, whereas in fact the selection pressure came from mefloquine use.

The mutation frequencies derived from *in vitro* studies are often much higher than those derived from observations *in vivo* (12). The absence of host defences and differences in antimalarial concentration profiles contribute to this discrepancy. The highest rates of emergence of resistance *in vivo* are for pyrimethamine and atovaquone. In the case of atovaquone, it has been estimated that one in three patients with symptomatic falciparum "contained", at presentation, a spontaneously arising atovaquone-resistant mutant parasite (5). For drugs such as chloroquine or artemisinin, the genetic events conferring resistance are much rarer. These genetic events may result in moderate changes in drug susceptibility, such that the drug still remains effective (e.g. as in the 108AsnDHFR mutation for pyrimethamine resistance) or, less commonly, very large reductions in susceptibility such that achievable concentrations of the drug are completely ineffective (e.g. as the cytochrome B mutations giving rise to atovaquone resistance) (13–16).

A6.3.3 Antimalarial pharmacokinetics and the selection of resistance

Absorption and disposition

The probability of selecting a *de novo* mutation that is resistant to antimalarials during the initial phase of treatment depends on the per-parasite frequency of the genetic event, the number of parasites present, immunity in the infected individual, and the relationship between the drug levels achieved and the degree of resistance conferred by the mutant parasite. Obviously, if the range of blood concentrations achieved in the patient considerably exceeds the concentrations giving 90% inhibition of multiplication (IC_{90} values) for the most resistant mutant (IC_{90}^R), then resistance cannot be selected in the acute phase of treatment as even the resistant mutants are prevented from multiplying. Conversely, if the degree of resistance provided by the genetic event is very small, the window of opportunity for selection may be negligible. Provided that there is such a window of selection then the broader the range of peak antimalarial concentrations and the closer the median value approaches IC_{90}^R, the greater the probability of selecting a resistant mutant in a patient. Peak drug concentrations are determined by absorption, distribution volume and dose. Several antimalarials (notably lumefantrine, halofantrine, atovaquone and, to a lesser extent, mefloquine) are lipophilic, hydrophobic and very variably absorbed (interindividual variation in bioavailability up to 20-fold) (17, 18). Interindividual variation in distribution volumes tends to be lower (usually less than five-fold) but, taken together with variable absorption, the outcome is considerable interindividual variation in peak antimalarial blood concentrations. The main sources of underdosing globally are incorrect self-medication because of poor adherence to the correctly prescribed drug regimen, poor quality drugs, uncontrolled drug availability and purchase of incorrect dose regimens, use of substandard drugs purchased in shops or markets, and incorrect administration in the home. The acute infection is the principal source of *de novo* resistance selection. Quality assured drugs, education, correct prescribing, good adherence, and optimized packaging and formulations therefore play pivotal roles in preventing the emergence of antimalarial drug resistance.

Drug elimination rates

In some areas of the world, transmission intensities may be as high as three infectious bites per person per day. In this context, a person who takes antimalarial treatment for symptomatic malaria exposes not only the parasites causing that infection to the drug, but also any newly acquired infections that emerge from the liver during the drug's elimination phase; the longer the terminal elimination half-life, the greater the exposure. The length of the terminal elimination half-life is an important determinant of the propensity for an antimalarial to select for resistance *(19–21)*. Some rapidly eliminated antimalarials (e.g. the artemisinin derivatives) never present an intermediate drug concentration to infecting malaria parasites because they are eliminated completely within the two-day life-cycle of the asexual parasite. Others (e.g. mefloquine, chloroquine) have elimination half-lives of weeks or months and present a lengthy selection opportunity.

With the exception of the artemisinin derivatives, maximum antimalarial parasite reduction ratios (kill rates) do not exceed 1000-fold per cycle *(22)*. Following hepatic schizogony, exposure of at least two asexual cycles (4 days) to therapeutic drug concentrations is therefore required to eradicate the blood stage parasites emerging from the liver. Even with maximum kill rates in the sensitive parasites and maximum growth rates in the resistant parasites, the resistant parasites only "overtake" the sensitive parasites in the third asexual cycle. Thus rapidly eliminated drugs (such as the artemisinin derivatives or quinine) cannot select during the elimination phase. Obviously, the greater the degree of resistance conferred by the resistance mutation – i.e. the higher the IC_{90}^R relative to the IC_{90} for susceptible parasites (IC_{90}^S) – the wider is the window of selection opportunity.

Patent gametocytaemia is more likely in recrudescent than in primary infections. Therefore, if *de novo* resistance arose in an acute symptomatic treated infection, the transmission probability from the subsequent recrudescent infection (bearing the new resistance genes) would be higher than from an infection newly acquired during the elimination phase of the antimalarial given for a previous infection, even if it attained the same parasite densities *(23)*.

A6.3.4 Spread of resistance

Several mathematical models have been devised to examine the spread of antimalarial drug resistance *(10, 21, 24, 25)*. Spread of resistance is determined by the reproductive advantage conferred by the resistance mechanism. This derives from the increased gametocyte carriage associated with treatment failure (both from the primary infection and the subsequent recrudescences) – the "donors", and then the selective pressure from residual concentrations of slowly eliminated antimalarial in potential recipients. A long elimination half-life results in long periods of post-treatment chemoprophylaxis.

Resistance encoded by multiple mutations at a single locus may be considered in two overlapping phases. The first phase, in which the drug is better tolerated by the parasites but therapeutic doses still usually clear the infection, and the second phase, when clinical failures start to occur. This second phase is very rapid and it is essential that surveillance programmes are in place and capable of monitoring the change from the first to the second phase. In areas of high transmission, the first phase may occur faster, but the subsequent phase slower. Combination therapy significantly slows the rate of evolution of resistance, but it should be instigated before significant resistance to either component is present.

A6.3.5 Prevention of resistance by use of combination therapy

The theory underlying combination treatment of tuberculosis, leprosy and HIV infection is well known, and has recently been applied to malaria *(4, 5, 24, 26–29)*. If two drugs with different modes of action, and therefore different resistance mechanisms, are used in combination, then the per-parasite probability of developing resistance to both drugs is the product of their individual per-parasite probabilities. For example, if the per-parasite probabilities of developing resistance to drug A and drug B are both 1 in 10^{12}, then a simultaneously resistant mutant will arise spontaneously in 1 in 10^{24} parasites. As it is postulated that there are approximately 10^{17} parasites in the entire world, and a cumulative total of less than 10^{20} in one year, such a simultaneously resistant parasite would arise spontaneously roughly once every 10 000 years – provided the drugs always confronted the parasites in combination. Thus the lower the *de novo* per-parasite probability of developing resistance, the greater the delay in the emergence of resistance.

Stable resistance to the artemisinin derivatives has not yet been identified, and cannot yet be induced in the laboratory, which suggests that it may be very rare indeed. *De novo* resistance to chloroquine is also very rare, and appears to have arisen and spread only twice in the world during the first decade of intensive use in the 1950s *(30)*. On the other hand, resistance to antifolate and atovaquone arises relatively frequently (e.g. antifolate resistance rose to high levels within two years of the initial deployment of proguanil in peninsular Malaya in 1947) and can be induced readily in experimental models (14, 27). Against a background of chloroquine resistance, mefloquine resistance arose over a six-year period on the north-west border of Thailand (31).

The ideal pharmacokinetic properties for an antimalarial have been much debated. Rapid elimination ensures that the residual concentrations do not provide a selective filter for resistant parasites, but drugs with this property (if used alone) must be given for at least 7 days, and adherence to 7-day regimens is poor. In order to be effective in a 3-day regimen, elimination half-lives usually need to exceed 24 h. Artemisinin derivatives are particularly effective in combinations with other antimalarials because of their very high killing rates (parasite reduction rate around 10 000-fold per cycle), lack of adverse effects and absence of significant resistance (5). Combinations of artemisinin derivatives (which are eliminated very rapidly) given for 3 days, with a slowly eliminated drug such as mefloquine, provide complete protection against the emergence of resistance to the artemisinin derivatives if adherence is good, but they do leave the slowly eliminated "tail" of mefloquine unprotected. Perhaps resistance could arise within the residual parasites that have not yet been killed by the artemisinin derivative. However, the number of parasites exposed to mefloquine alone is a tiny fraction (less than 0.00001%) of those present in the acute symptomatic infection. Furthermore, these residual parasites "see" relatively high levels of mefloquine and, even if susceptibility was reduced, these levels may be sufficient to eradicate the infection (Figure A6.2). The long mefloquine tail does, however, provide a selective filter for resistant parasites acquired from elsewhere, and therefore contributes to the spread of resistance once it has developed. Yet on the north-west border of Thailand, an area of low transmission where mefloquine resistance had already developed, systematic deployment of the artesunate-mefloquine combination was dramatically effective in stopping resistance and also in reducing the incidence of malaria (31, 32). This strategy is thought to be effective at preventing the emergence of resistance at higher levels of transmission, where high-biomass infections still constitutes the major source of de novo resistance.

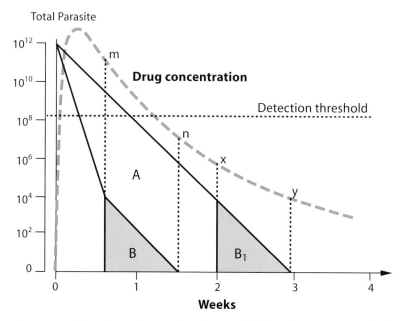

Total Parasite

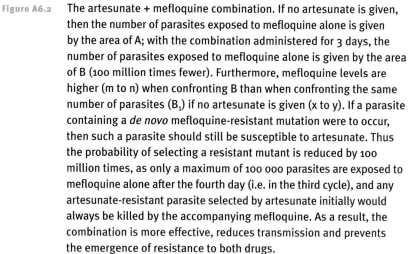

Figure A6.2   The artesunate + mefloquine combination. If no artesunate is given, then the number of parasites exposed to mefloquine alone is given by the area of A; with the combination administered for 3 days, the number of parasites exposed to mefloquine alone is given by the area of B (100 million times fewer). Furthermore, mefloquine levels are higher (m to n) when confronting B than when confronting the same number of parasites (B₁) if no artesunate is given (x to y). If a parasite containing a *de novo* mefloquine-resistant mutation were to occur, then such a parasite should still be susceptible to artesunate. Thus the probability of selecting a resistant mutant is reduced by 100 million times, as only a maximum of 100 000 parasites are exposed to mefloquine alone after the fourth day (i.e. in the third cycle), and any artesunate-resistant parasite selected by artesunate initially would always be killed by the accompanying mefloquine. As a result, the combination is more effective, reduces transmission and prevents the emergence of resistance to both drugs.

A6.4   A summary of the global distribution of antimalarial drug resistance

Resistance to antimalarials has been a particular problem with *P. falciparum*, in which widespread resistance to chloroquine, sulfadoxine-pyrimethamine and mefloquine has been observed (Figure A6.3). Antifolate and chloroquine resistance has developed in *P. vivax* in several areas, and chloroquine resistance in *P. malariae* has also recently been reported. No significant resistance has yet been observed to artemisinin and its derivatives despite their extensive deployment in several parts of Asia.

Malaria transmission areas and reported *P. falciparum* resistance, 2004

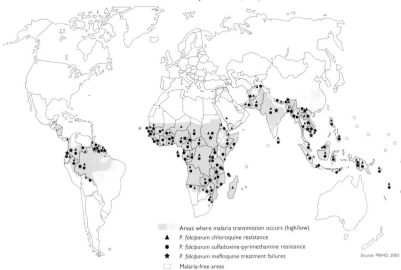

Areas where malaria transmission occurs (high/low)
▲ *P. falciparum* chloroquine resistance
● *P. falciparum* sulfadoxine-pyrimethamine resistance
★ *P. falciparum* mefloquine treatment failures
☐ Malaria-free areas

Source: ©WHO, 2005

Figure A6.3   Malaria transmission areas and the distribution of reported resistance or treatment failures with selected antimalarial drugs, September 2004 (mefloquine resistance in Africa is currently being further reviewed)

A6.4.1 *Plasmodium falciparum* resistance

Chloroquine

The first reports of chloroquine resistance occurred in Thailand and Colombia in the late 1950s, around 12 years after the drug's introduction. By 1980, all endemic areas in South America were affected, and by 1989, most of Asia and Oceania. In Africa, chloroquine resistance emerged in 1978 in the east, and gradually spread westwards through the 1980s. Resistance has now been documented in all falciparum-endemic areas except Central America and the Caribbean *(33)*. Recent molecular studies favour importation of chloroquine resistance to Africa from East Asia *(34, 35)*. Chloroquine resistance has emerged independently less than ten times in the past 50 years (Figure A6.4).

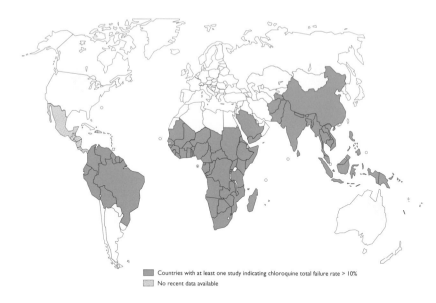

Countries with at least one study indicating chloroquine total failure rate > 10%
No recent data available

Figure A6.4 **Distribution of chloroquine resistance in *Plasmodium falciparum***

Sulfadoxine-pyrimethamine

Resistance to pyrimethamine emerged rapidly after its deployment for treatment, prophylaxis and, in some areas, mass treatment in the 1950s. Resistance to both components of sulfadoxine-pyrimethamine was noted shortly after this drug was introduced over a decade later. In South-East Asia this occurred on the Thai-Cambodian border in the mid-1960s. Resistance became an operational problem in the same area within the few years of the introduction of sulfadoxine-pyrimethamine to the malaria control programme in 1975 *(36)*. High-level resistance is found in many parts of South-East Asia, southern China and the Amazon basin, and lower levels of resistance are seen on the coast of South America and in southern Asia and Oceania. In eastern Africa, sulfadoxine-pyrimethamine sensitivity was observed to be declining in the 1980s and resistance has progressed westwards across Africa relentlessly over the last decade. Clinical failure rates of more than 25% have already been reported in Liberia *(37)*, Guinea Bissau *(38)* and Malawi *(39)*.

Many areas now have high-level resistance with high-treatment failure rates in children. Recent molecular evidence suggests a common South-East Asian origin of the resistant *P. falciparum* parasites now prevalent in much of southern and Central Africa (triple *dhfr* mutant) *(9, 40–42)* (Figure A6.5).

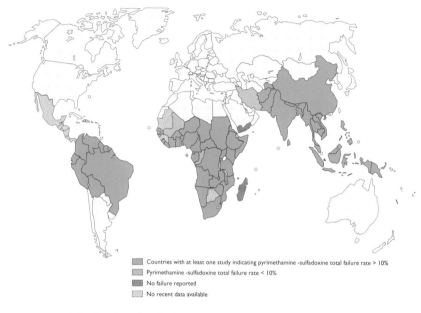

Countries with at least one study indicating pyrimethamine -sulfadoxine total failure rate > 10%
Pyrimethamine -sulfadoxine total failure rate < 10%
No failure reported
No recent data available

Figure A6.5   Distribution of sulfadoxine-pyrimethamine resistance in
               Plasmodium falciparum

Mefloquine

Mefloquine resistance was first observed on the Thai-Cambodian and Thai-
Burmese borders in the late 1980s *(43, 44)* and the monotherapy is no longer
effective there. Migrant gem miners returning from Cambodia may have been
the means of spread of mefloquine resistance to India and Bangladesh *(45)*.
Isolated cases of mefloquine resistance have also been reported from the
Amazon basin, and *in vitro* studies in Africa have identified some *P. falciparum*
strains with low mefloquine sensitivity. Overall, clinical mefloquine resistance
outside South-East Asia is rare (Figure A6.6).

The main determinant of mefloquine resistance is amplification of the gene
(*Pfmdr*) that encodes the multidrug transporter *(46)*. Amplification occurs
only for the "wild type" allele explaining the inverse relationship between
sensitivity to chloroquine (the *Pfmdr* Tyr86 mutation is associated with
reduced sensitivity) and to mefloquine (and to the structurally related drugs,
quinine and halofantrine) *(15)*.

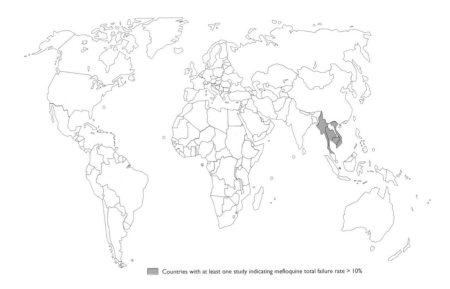

Countries with at least one study indicating mefloquine total failure rate > 10%

Figure A6.6   **Distribution of mefloquine resistance in *Plasmodium falciparum***

Quinine

The first reports of possible quinine resistance occurred in Brazil almost 100 years ago. Even today, however, clinical resistance to quinine monotherapy is reported only sporadically in South-East Asia and western Oceania, and resistance in Africa and South America is much less frequent. Widespread use of quinine in Thailand in the 1980 s led to significant reduction in its sensitivity *(45)*. Quinine is therefore now used in combination with an antibiotic, usually tetracycline, doxycycline or clindamycin, and is reserved for cases of severe malaria. *Pfmdr1* mutations associated with chloroquine resistance have been believed to be associated with reduced susceptibility to quinine *(47, 48)*.

Artemisinin

Except in an animal model, there have been no confirmed reports of artemisinin resistance in malaria parasites that infect humans. The pharmacological characteristics of the drug, namely short elimination half-life, rapidity of action and ability to reduce gametocyte carriage, should delay the onset of significant resistance. Artemisinin derivatives are associated with high recrudescence rates (~10%) after monotherapy, so are usually combined with longer-acting antimalarials for clinical treatment. These recrudescences, however, are not a result of resistance.

Multidrug resistance

Multidrug resistance is generally defined as resistance to three or more antimalarial compounds from different chemical classes. Generally, the first two classes are 4-aminoquinolines (e.g. chloroquine) and antifolates (e.g. sulfadoxine-pyrimethamine). The precise amount of resistance needed in order for a drug to be considered as failing is not universally agreed. Some consider clinical cure rates of less than 75% to be the minimum required for classification as failure, while the current recommendations aim for cure rates over 90%.

Established multidrug resistance occurs in South-East Asia (particularly along the borders of Thailand with Burma and Cambodia) and in the Amazon basin. In Thailand, mefloquine monotherapy was replaced with the combination of high-dose mefloquine and artesunate given for 3 days. Mefloquine resistance has been reduced by the use of this combination, as cure rates of more than 95% have been sustained for over 10 years, and susceptibility to mefloquine has actually improved despite extensive deployment of the combination.

Several areas are at risk of multidrug resistance, as resistance to chloroquine and sulfadoxine-pyrimethamine is already widespread. Progressive loss of sulfadoxine-pyrimethamine efficacy should be taken as a warning sign.

A6.4.2 *Plasmodium vivax* resistance

Chloroquine

Resistance of *P. vivax* is rare and generally limited to chloroquine resistance, which was first reported in the late 1980s in Papua New Guinea and Indonesia. Focal true chloroquine resistance (with whole blood chloroquine + desethylchloroquine concentrations of >100 ng/ml on the day of failure) or prophylactic and/or treatment failure not necessarily related to true resistance, have since also been observed in Brazil, Colombia, Ethiopia, Guatemala, Guyana, India, Republic of Korea, Myanmar, Solomon Islands, Thailand and Turkey.

A6.4.3 *Plasmodium malariae* resistance

Chloroquine

Resistance of *P. malariae* to chloroquine was observed recently in Indonesia.

A6.5 Monitoring of antimalarial drug resistance

A6.5.1 Monitoring methods

The rapid spread of antimalarial drug resistance over the last few decades has increased the need for monitoring, in order to ensure proper management of clinical cases, allow for early detection of changing patterns of resistance, and suggest where national malaria treatment policies should be revised. The monitoring procedures available include therapeutic efficacy testing (also known as *in vivo* testing). This involves the repeated assessment of clinical and parasitological outcomes of treatment – during a fixed period of follow-up – in order to detect any reappearance of symptoms and signs of clinical malaria and/or parasites in the blood, which would indicate reduced parasite sensitivity with the particular drug. Other methods include *in vitro* studies of parasite susceptibility to drugs in culture, and studies of point mutations or duplications in parasite resistance genes with molecular methods (polymerase chain reaction, PCR). Animal models are also used, although not routinely.

In vivo tests

(a) Therapeutic efficacy testing and the WHO standard protocol for P. falciparum

From a programmatic point of view, data on therapeutic efficacy are most useful in deciding whether or not a drug is still appropriate as first-line treatment. Therapeutic efficacy studies are relatively simple to conduct, and the requirements in terms of training of staff and technical facilities are therefore limited. However, the results can be affected by misdiagnosis and incorrect drug administration. In order to interpret and allow for comparison of the results within and between regions, and to follow trends over time, studies need to be conducted according to similar procedures and standards. WHO therefore recommends the use of the WHO standard protocol, which provides guidance on how best to obtain the minimum necessary information about the therapeutic responses to an antimalarial so as to allow informed decision-making on its future use *(49)*.

The protocol is designed for use in the assessment of antimalarial drugs or drug combinations used routinely for treatment of uncomplicated *P. falciparum* malaria (chloroquine, sulfadoxine-pyrimethamine, amodiaquine, artemisinin-based combination therapies and others). It comprises a simple, one-arm prospective evaluation of clinical and parasitological treatment responses in children aged 6–59 months, in whom the level of acquired immunity is relatively low and therefore has only a minor influence on the outcome of the test. To ensure a reasonable specificity of the malaria diagnosis in areas of intense transmission, only individuals with a parasite density ≥ 2000 asexual parasites/μl of blood should be included in studies. In areas of low to moderate transmission, individuals with ≥ 1000 asexual parasites/μl can be included. Further methodological and operational considerations in relation to case definition, sample size calculations, ethical concerns and the criteria for inclusion and exclusion, some of which some relate only to specific drugs, are explained in detail in the protocol.

The recommended duration of follow-up is ≥ 28 days in areas of intense as well as low to moderate transmission. As a significant proportion of treatment failures do not appear until after day 14, shorter observation periods lead to a considerable overestimation of the efficacy of the tested drug. This is a particular problem at low levels of resistance and with low failure rates (50). As the objective of treatment is cure of the infection, and cure rates of more than 90% are required, the cure rate must be adequately characterized. For relatively effective, slowly eliminated antimalarials, half the recrudescences may occur after 28 days. For treatment with drugs such as amodiaquine, chloroquine and sulfadoxine-pyrimethamine, a 28-day follow-up is considered appropriate; follow-up periods of 42 days and 63 days are recommended for artemether-lumefantrine and mefloquine, respectively (51). These follow-up periods will capture most but often not all recrudescent infections – particularly at low levels of resistance. Studies even of > 28 days of duration risk loss to follow-up and should be accompanied by molecular assessments (PCR genotyping) so as to distinguish recrudescence from reinfection. If surveillance programmes do not have access to molecular techniques, studies of 14 days of duration without PCR adjustments can still provide useful information on failing drugs (i.e. to justify their replacement) – but they cannot be used to justify inclusion or continued recommendation. In areas of low to moderate transmission, the use of molecular methods is recommended, but is not strictly essential if the likelihood of reinfection is relatively small. PCR genotyping involves comparison of polymorphic parasite genes, usually those encoding variable blocks within PfMSP2, and also sometimes PfMSP1 and PfGLURP, in whole blood samples taken during the acute and recurrent infections.

The WHO standard protocol classifies outcomes of efficacy studies into the following four categories: early treatment failure, late clinical failure, late parasitological failure, and adequate clinical and parasitological response. These classifications rely on the presence or absence of fever or other signs of clinical malaria and/or presence of parasitaemia during the course of follow-up (Table A6.1). The therapeutic response is classified as early treatment failure if the patient develops clinical or parasitological symptoms during the first 3 days of follow-up. The response is classified as late clinical failure if symptoms develop during the follow-up period (from day 4 to day 28), without previously meeting the criteria for early treatment failure. It is a late parasitological failure if only parasitaemia reappear without any symptom, in the period from day 7 to day 28. Adequate clinical and parasitological response is defined as the absence of symptoms and of parasitaemia on day 28, without any of the criteria for the other three categories having been met previously.

Table A6.1 **Classification of treatment outcomes in studies of antimalarial drug efficacy in areas of low, moderate and intense transmission** *(49)*

Treatment outcome	Symptoms and signs
Early treatment failure	• Development of danger signs or severe malaria on days 1–3 in the presence of parasitaemia • Parasitaemia on day 2 higher than the day 0 count irrespective of axillary temperature • Parasitaemia on day 3 with axillary temperature $\geq 37.5\ ^\circ C$ • Parasitaemia on day 3 that is $\geq 25\%$ of count on day 0.
Late treatment failure	
• Late clinical failure	• Development of danger signs or severe malaria after day 3 in the presence of parasitaemia, without previously meeting any of the criteria of early treatment failure • Presence of parasitaemia and axillary temperature $\geq 37.5\ ^\circ C$ (or history of fever) on any day from day 4 to day 28, without previously meeting any of the criteria of early treatment failure.
• Late parasitological failure	• Presence of parasitaemia on any day from day 7 to day 28 and axillary temperature $< 37.5\ ^\circ C$, without previously meeting any of the criteria of early treatment failure or late clinical failure.
Adequate clinical and parasitological response	• Absence of parasitaemia on day 28 irrespective of axillary temperature without previously meeting any of the criteria of early treatment failure, late clinical failure or late parasitological failure.

For simplicity, the outcome of efficacy studies can be summarized as "clinical failure", which is equal to the sum of early treatment failure and late clinical failure, and as "total failure", which is equal to the sum of early treatment failure, late clinical failure and late parasitological failure. The rates of clinical failure and total failure are used to define cut-off points for drug policy change, using the standard WHO protocol. It should be noted that the most recent classification of therapeutic responses described above differs from that used previously; late parasitological treatment responses are now also considered as an indicator of drug efficacy, as persistent parasitaemia is associated with increased risk of clinical malaria, anaemia and increased gametocyte carriage *(52)*. The protocol provides guidance on how to calculate and present efficacy test results.

If feasible, any judgement of the therapeutic efficacy of a drug should be accompanied by measurements of blood drug concentrations, to ensure that therapeutic drug levels were reached; subtherapeutic levels confound the efficacy result. With modern techniques, antimalarial drug concentrations can often be analysed in small samples of blood dried on filter paper; samples can be sent to a central pharmacological laboratory for analysis.

(b) In vivo *assessment of resistance in* P. malariae
Protocols similar to those used for *P. falciparum* can be used.

(c) In vivo *assessment of resistance in* P. vivax *and* P. ovale *infections*
Relapse and recrudescence cannot be distinguished reliably in these infections, as they will usually have the same genotype. Nevertheless the *in vivo* assessment of chloroquine susceptibility can be performed using the same format as for *P. falciparum*, with a follow-up period of 28 or preferably 35 days, and preferably accompanied by measurement of whole blood chloroquine and desethychloroquine levels. Recurrent infections within this period presenting with whole blood chloroquine + desethychloroquine concentrations exceeding 100 ng/ml can be considered as resistant whether they are a relapse, a recrudescence, or even a new infection, as this concentration should be suppressive *(50, 53, 54)*.

In vitro resistance tests

To support evidence of a failing antimalarial, *in vitro* tests can be used to provide a more accurate measure of drug sensitivity under controlled experimental conditions. Parasites obtained from finger-prick blood are placed in microtitre wells, exposed to precisely known concentrations of a particular drug and examined for the inhibition of maturation into schizont parasite stages *(55)*. This test overcomes some of the many confounding factors influencing the results of *in vivo* tests, such as subtherapeutic drug concentrations and the influence of host factors on parasite growth (e.g. factors related to acquired immunity), and therefore provide a more accurate picture of the "true" level of resistance to the drug. Multiple tests can be performed on parasite isolates, using several drugs and drug combinations simultaneously. New experimental drugs can also be tested in this way. However, partly because *in vitro* tests do not include host factors, the correlation between results of *in vitro* and *in vivo* tests is not consistent and is not well understood. Furthermore, different parasite isolates may adapt differently to culture, which may affect the test result. For example, if a resistant strain adapts less well to culture and therefore dies off earlier, the outcome is an overestimation of its susceptibility. Prodrugs such as proguanil, which require conversion into active metabolites in the human host, cannot be tested, and *P. vivax, P. ovale* and *P. malariae* cannot be evaluated *in vitro* owing to constraints in culturing these species (although this has now largely been overcome for *P. vivax*). *In vitro* testing is more demanding in terms of technology and resources, and is not ideal for routine drug efficacy evaluation under field conditions. It should therefore primarily be used to provide additional information to support clinical efficacy data at selected resistance-monitoring sites.

Molecular markers

In recent years, molecular tests have been developed for the detection of parasite gene mutations or amplifications associated with resistance to antimalarials as an additional means of assessing levels of drug resistance. These methods are based on PCR, using small amounts of parasite DNA material in finger-prick blood dried on filter paper.

Information on the prevalence of gene mutations may give an indication of the level of drug resistance in an area, and relatively well-defined molecular markers of resistance have been established for pyrimethamine (*Pfdhfr* and *Pvdhfr*), sulfadoxine (*Pfdhps*) and chloroquine (*Pfcrt1*) (56, 57). Amplification of *Pfmdr* (for mefloquine resistance) is considerably more technically demanding, requiring validated real-time PCR. No markers are yet available for other antimalarials.

These methods have their disadvantages. The results are seldom available rapidly, and mutations and the measured therapeutic efficacy do not always correlate well, as many factors determine the therapeutic response in addition to parasite sensitivity to the antimalarial drug treatment. However, serial assessment of molecular markers can be a useful guide to the emergence of resistance, especially if used consistently over time in comparable study populations to detect trends. The methods may also provide useful guidance on choices of treatment during acute malaria epidemics, where time will not allow for clinical efficacy tests, but where it may be critical to avoid the use of a particular drug (58). The requirements for technical skills and laboratory facilities prevent the routine use of these methods in most drug efficacy testing sites, although they are becoming increasingly used in laboratories in endemic areas – particularly those supporting clinical trials. Moreover, the results are subject to error and must be considered carefully. For example, a patient may have an infection with two different genotypes on day 0 but, only one genotype is detected with PCR. If one genotype is sensitive and the other is resistant, the resistant genotype may persist until day 14 despite antimalarial treatment, while the sensitive genotype will be cleared; if detected, the presence of the resistant genotype on day 14 may then incorrectly be interpreted as reinfection and not as recrudescence *(59)*.

While monitoring of molecular markers may only be possible at central laboratories, it can support monitoring programmes that rely on *in vivo* testing, and also play an important part in early-warning systems to guide treatment policies coordinated at national and regional levels. With newly developed high-throughput methods *(60, 61)*, more comprehensive population-based analyses will also be possible, which may allow for a better understanding and prediction of the future spread of resistance *(40, 42)*.

Efficacy testing in animal models

In addition to *in vivo* efficacy studies involving human participants, drug sensitivity can be tested in animal models. Although such models do not play an important role in routine efficacy-monitoring programmes, they may be useful in the testing of newly developed drugs, not yet approved for use in humans, or to minimize the influence of host immunity on drug efficacy, while retaining the influence of some of the extrinsic factors observed in *in vivo* studies.

A6.5.2   Reporting of treatment failures

Reports of cases of treatment failure and decreased drug sensitivity have often provided important first evidence for more widespread resistance in an area. Although such evidence is subject to bias, it can be collected without much effort at peripheral health centres. If standardized and registered, such reports can make a valuable contribution to national early-warning systems, facilitating cost-effective monitoring by national programmes.

A6.5.3   Criteria for antimalarial drug policy change

The *WHO malaria treatment guidelines* recommend that antimalarial treatment policy should be changed at treatment failure rates considerably lower than those recommended previously. This major change reflects the availability of highly effective drugs, and the recognition both of the consequences of drug resistance, in terms of morbidity and mortality, and of the importance of high cure rates in malaria control.

It is now recommended that a change of first-line treatment should be initiated if the total failure proportion exceeds 10%. However, it is acknowledged that a decision to change may be influenced by a number of other factors, including the prevalence and geographical distribution of reported treatment failures, health service provider and/or patient dissatisfaction with the treatment, political and economical contexts, and the availability of affordable alternatives to the commonly used treatment.

A6.6   References

1. Bonhoeffer S, Lipsitch M, Levin BR. Evaluating treatment protocols to prevent antibiotic resistance. *Proceedings of the National Academy of Sciences of the USA*, 1997, 94:12106–12111.

2. Lipsitch M, Levin BR. The population dynamics of antimicrobial chemotherapy. *Antimicrobial Agents and Chemotherapy*, 1997, 41:363–373.

3. Austin DJ, Anderson RM. Studies of antibiotic resistance within the patient, hospitals and the community using simple mathematical models. *Philosophical Transactions of the Royal Society of London, Series B, Biological Sciences*, 1999, 354:721–738.

4. Peters W. *Chemotherapy and drug resistance in malaria*, 2nd ed. London, Academic Press, 1987.

5. White NJ. Antimalarial drug resistance and combination chemotherapy. *Philosophical Transactions of the Royal Society of London, Series B, Biological Sciences*, 1999, 354:739–749.

6. Jeffery GM, Eyles DE. Infectivity to mosquitoes of *Plasmodium falciparum* as related to gametocyte density and duration of infection. *American Journal of Tropical Medicine and Hygiene*, 1955, 4:781–789.

7. Mackinnon MJ, Hastings IM. The evolution of multiple drug resistance in malaria parasites. *Transactions of the Royal Society of Tropical Medicine and Hygiene*, 1998, 92:188–195.

8. Hastings IM, Mackinnon MJ. The emergence of drug-resistant malaria. *Parasitology*, 1998, 117:411–417.

9. Roper C et al. Intercontinental spread of pyrimethamine-resistant malaria. *Science*, 2004, 305:1124.

10. Dye C, Williams BG. Multigenic drug resistance among inbred malaria parasites. *Proceedings of the Royal Society of London, Series B, Biological Sciences*, 1997, 264: 61–67.

11. Gatton ML, Martin LB, Cheng Q. Evolution of resistance to sulfadoxine-pyrimethamine in *Plasmodium falciparum*. *Antimicrobial Agents and Chemotherapy*, 2004, 48:2116–2123.

12. Rathod PK, McErlean T, Lee PC. Variations in frequencies of drug resistance in *Plasmodium falciparum*. *Proceedings of the National Academy of Sciences of the USA*, 1997, 94:9389–9393.

13. Cowman AF, Galatis D, Thompson JK. Selection for mefloquine resistance in *Plasmodium falciparum* is linked to amplification of the *pfmdr1* gene and cross-resistance to halofantrine and quinine. *Proceedings of the National Academy of Sciences of the USA*, 1994, 91:1143–1147.

14. Looareesuwan S et al. Clinical studies of atovaquone, alone or in combination with other antimalarial drugs, for treatment of acute uncomplicated malaria in Thailand. *American Journal of Tropical Medicine and Hygiene*, 1996, 54:62–66.

15. Reed MB et al. *Pgh1* modulates sensitivity and resistance to multiple antimalarials in *Plasmodium falciparum*. *Nature*, 2000, 403: 906–909.

16. Korsinczky M. et al. Mutations in *Plasmodium falciparum* cytochrome b that are associated with atovaquone resistance are located at a putative drug-binding site. *Antimicrobial Agents and Chemotherapy*, 2000, 44: 2100–2108.

17. White NJ. Antimalarial pharmacokinetics and treatment regimens. *British Journal of Clinical Pharmacology*, 1992, 34:1–10.

18. White NJ, van Vugt M, Ezzet F. Clinical pharmacokinetics and pharmacodynamics of artemether-lumefantrine. *Clinical Pharmacokinetics*, 1999, 37:105–125.

19. Watkins WM, Mosobo M. Treatment of *Plasmodium falciparum* malaria with pyrimethamine-sulphadoxine: selective pressure for resistance is a function of long elimination half-life. *Transactions of the Royal Society of Tropical Medicine and Hygiene*, 1973, 87:75–78.

20. Nzila AM et al. Molecular evidence of greater selective pressure for drug resistance exerted by the long-acting antifolate Pyrimethamine/Sulfadoxine compared with the shorter-acting chlorproguanil/dapsone on Kenyan *Plasmodium falciparum*. *Journal of Infectious Diseases*, 2000, 181:2023–2028.

21. Hastings I, Watkins WM, White NJ. The evolution of drug-resistance in malaria: the role of the terminal elimination half-life. *Philosophical Transactions of the Royal Society London B Biological Sciences*, 2002, 357:505–519.

22. White NJ. Assessment of the pharmacodynamic properties of antimalarial drugs in vivo. *Antimicrobial Agents and Chemotherapy*, 1997, 41: 1413–1422.

23. Price RN et al. Risk factors for gametocyte carriage in uncomplicated falciparum malaria. *American Journal of Tropical Medicine and Hygiene,* 1999, 60: 1019–1023.

24. Curtis CF, Otoo LN. A simple model of the build-up of resistance to mixtures of antimalarial drugs. *Transactions of the Royal Society of Tropical Medicine and Hygiene*, 1986, 80: 889–892.

25. Hastings IM. The origins of antimalarial drug resistance. *Trends in Parasitology*, 2004, 20:512–518.

26. Peters W. Drug resistance – a perspective. *Transactions of the Royal Society of Tropical Medicine and Hygiene*, 1969, 63:25–45.

27. Peters W. The prevention of antimalarial drug resistance. *Pharmacology and Therapeutics*, 1990, 47:499–508.

28. Chawira AN et al. The effect of combinations of qinghaosu (artemisinin) with standard antimalarial drugs in the suppressive treatment of malaria in mice. *Transactions of the Royal Society of Tropical Medicine and Hygiene*, 1987, 81:554–558.

29. White NJ et al. Averting a malaria disaster. *Lancet*, 1999, 353:1965–1967.

30. Su, X et al. Complex polymorphisms in an approximately 330 kDa protein are linked to chloroquine-resistant *P. falciparum* in Southeast Asia and Africa. *Cell*, 1997, 91: 593–603.

31. Nosten F et al. Effects of artesunate-mefloquine combination on incidence of *Plasmodium falciparum* malaria and mefloquine resistance in western Thailand; a prospective study. *Lancet*, 2000, 356: 297–302.

32. Brockman A et al. *Plasmodium falciparum* antimalarial drug susceptibility on the northwestern border of Thailand during five years of extensive artesunate-mefloquine use. *Transactions of the Royal Society of Tropical Medicine and Hygiene*, 2000, 94, 537–544.

33. Wongsrichanalai C et al. Epidemiology of drug-resistant malaria. *Lancet Infectious Diseases*, 2002, 2:209–218.

34. Wellems TE, Plowe CV. Chloroquine-resistant malaria. *Journal of Infectious Diseases*, 2001, 184:770–776.

35. Vieira PP et al. pfcrt Polymorphism and the spread of chloroquine resistance in *Plasmodium falciparum* populations across the Amazon Basin. *Journal of Infectious Diseases*, 2004, 190:417–424.

36. Hurwitz ES, Johnson D, Campbell CC. Resistance of *Plasmodium falciparum* malaria to sulfadoxine-pyrimethamine ("Fansidar") in a refugee camp in Thailand. *Lancet*, 1981, 1:1068–1070.

37. Checchi F et al. High *Plasmodium falciparum* resistance to chloroquine and sulfadoxine-pyrimethamine in Harper, Liberia: results in vivo and analysis of point mutations. *Transactions of the Royal Society of Tropical Medicine and Hygiene*, 2002, 96:664–669.

38. Kofoed PE et al. Treatment of uncomplicated malaria in children in Guinea-Bissau with chloroquine, quinine, and sulfadoxine-pyrimethamine. *Transactions of the Royal Society of Tropical Medicine and Hygiene*, 2002, 96:304–309.

39. Plowe CV et al. Sustained clinical efficacy of sulfadoxine-pyrimethamine for uncomplicated falciparum malaria in Malawi after 10 years as first line treatment: five year prospective study. *British Medical Journal*, 2004, 328:545.

40. Anderson TJ. Mapping drug resistance genes in *Plasmodium falciparum* by genome-wide association. *Current Drug Targets. Infectious Disorders*, 2004, 4:65–78.

41. Nair S et al. A selective sweep driven by pyrimethamine treatment in southeast Asian malaria parasites. *Molecular Biology and Evolution*, 2003, 20:1526–1536.

42. Roper C et al. Antifolate antimalarial resistance in southeast Africa: a population-based analysis. *Lancet*, 2003, 361:1174–1181.

43. Nosten F et al. Mefloquine-resistant falciparum malaria on the Thai-Burmese border. *Lancet*, 1991, 337:1140–1143.

44. Fontanet AL et al. High prevalence of mefloquine-resistant falciparum malaria in eastern Thailand. *Bulletin of the World Health Organization*, 1993, 71:377–383.

45. Wernsdorfer WH. Epidemiology of drug resistance in malaria. *Acta Tropica*, 1994, 56:143–156.

46. Price RN et al. Mefloquine resistance in *Plasmodium falciparum* and increased pfmdr1 gene copy number. *Lancet*, 2004, 364:438–447.

47. Zalis MG et al. Characterization of *Plasmodium falciparum* isolated from the Amazon region of Brazil: evidence for quinine resistance. *American Journal of Tropical Medicine and Hygiene*, 1998, 58:630–637.

48. Duraisingh MT et al. Linkage disequilibrium between two chromosomally distinct loci associated with increased resistance to chloroquine in *Plasmodium falciparum*. *Parasitology*, 2000, 121:1–7.

49. *Assessment and monitoring of antimalarial drug efficacy for the treatment of uncomplicated falciparum malaria*. Geneva, World Health Organization, 2003 (document WHO/HTM/RBM/2003.50).

50. White NJ. The assessment of antimalarial drug efficacy. *Trends in Parasitology*, 2002, 18: 458–464.

51. Ringwald P. Monitoring antimalarial drug efficacy. *Clinical Infectious Diseases*, 2004, 38:1192-1193.

52. *Assessment of therapeutic efficacy of antimalarial drugs for uncomplicated falciparum malaria in areas with intense transmission*. Geneva, World Health Organization, 1996 (document WHO/MAL/96.1077).

53. Baird JK et al. Diagnosis of resistance to chloroquine by *Plasmodium vivax*: timing of recurrence and whole blood chloroquine levels. *American Journal of Tropical Medicine and Hygiene*, 1997, 56:621–626.

54. Baird JK. Chloroquine resistance in *Plasmodium vivax*. *Antimicrobial Agents and Chemotherapy*, 2004, 48:4075–4083.

55. Rieckmann K.H. et al. Drug sensitivity of *Plasmodium falciparum*. An in-vitro microtechnique. *Lancet*, 1978, 1:22–23.

56. Djimde A et al. A molecular marker for chloroquine-resistant falciparum malaria. *New England Journal of Medicine*, 2001, 344:257–263.

57. Kublin J.G. et al. Molecular markers for failure of sulfadoxine-pyrimethamine and chlorproguanil-dapsone treatment of *Plasmodium falciparum* malaria. *Journal of Infectious Diseases*, 2002, 185:380–388.

58. Djimde A et al. Molecular diagnosis of resistance to antimalarial drugs during epidemics and in war zones. *Journal of Infectious Diseases*, 2004, 190:853–855.

59. Snounou G, Beck HP. The use of PCR genotyping in the assessment of recrudescence or reinfection after antimalarial drug treatment. *Parasitology Today*, 1998, 14:462–467.

60. Pearce RJ et al. Molecular determination of point mutation haplotypes in the dihydrofolate reductase and dihydropteroate synthase of *Plasmodium falciparum* in three districts of northern Tanzania. *Antimicrobial Agents and Chemotherapy*, 2003, 47:1347–1354.

61. Alifrangis A et al. A simple high-throughput method to detect *P. falciparum* single nucleotide polymorphisms in the dihydrofolate reductase, dihydropterate synthase, and *P. falciparum* chloroquine resistance transporter genes using polymerase chain reaction- and enzyme-linked immunosorbent assay-based technology. *American Journal of Tropical Medicine and Hygiene*, 2005, 72:155–162.

Annex 7.   Uncomplicated *P. falciparum* malaria

ANNEX 7

UNCOMPLICATED *P. FALCIPARUM* MALARIA

A7.1 How do artemisinin combination therapies compare with non-artemisinin monotherapies?

Systematic review and meta-analysis of individual patient data from 16 randomized trials (total of 5948 people) that studied the effects of the addition of artesunate to monotherapy for falciparum malaria *(1)* (search date, September 2002). The analysis compared odds ratios (OR) of parasitological failure at days 14 and 28 (artesunate combination compared to monotherapy) and calculated combined summary ORs across trials using standard methods. Results comprise parasite failure including re-infections by day 28 in 14 trials (Figure A7.1), and parasite failure excluding re-infections in 11 trials (Figure A7.2).

Review: Artesunate combination treatments for malaria
Comparison: 01 Artesunate combinations versus no artesunate
Outcome: 02 Parasitaemia by day 28 (all)

Study or sub-category	Treatment n/N	Control n/N	OR (fixed) 95% CI	OR (fixed) 95% CI	Quality
02 Amodiaquine					
Gabon	14/94	28/98		0.44 [0.21, 0.90]	D
Ken_AMRF	57/180	108/183		0.32 [0.21, 0.50]	D
Senegal	29/159	33/156		0.83 [0.48, 1.45]	D
Subtotal (95% CI)	433	437		0.46 [0.34, 0.62]	
Total events: 100 (Treatment), 169 (Control)					
Test for hetetogeneity: Chi² = 7.01, df = 2(P = 0.03), I² = 71.5%					
Test for overall effect: Z = 5.06 (P < 0.00001)					
03 Sulfadoxine-pyrimethamine					
Gambia	6/187	20/193		0.29 [0.11, 0.73]	D
Ken_KMRI	89/192	121/189		0.49 [0.32, 0.73]	D
Ken_W	52/189	107/189		0.29 [0.19, 0.45]	D
Malawi	41/134	99/129		0.13 [0.08, 0.23]	D
Peru	2/97	4/93		0.47 [0.08, 2.62]	D
Uganda	48/116	89/144		0.44 [0.26, 0.72]	D
Subtotal (95% CI)	915	937		0.32 [0.26, 0.40]	
Total events: 238 (Treatment), 440 (Control)					
Test for hetetogeneity: Chi² = 15.56, df = 5(P = 0.008), I² = 67.9%					
Test for overall effect: Z = 10.05 (P < 0.00001)					
04 Mefloquine					
Thai-2	1/180	46/169		0.01 [0.00, 0.11]	D
Thai-3	9/179	57/181		0.12 [0.05, 0.24]	D
Subtotal (95% CI)	359	350		0.07 [0.03, 0.13]	
Total events: 10 (Treatment), 103 (Control)					
Test for hetetogeneity: Chi² = 4.14, df = 1(P = 0.04), I² = 75.9%					
Test for overall effect: Z = 7.80 (P < 0.00001)					
Total (95% CI)	1707	1724		0.30 [0.26, 0.36]	
Total events: 348 (Treatment), 712 (Control)					
Test for hetetogeneity: Chi² = 44.83, df = 10(P = 0.04), I² = 77.7%					
Test for overall effect: Z = 13.80 (P < 0.00001)					

0.01   0.1   1   10   100
Favours treatment   Favours control

df, degrees of freedom; OR: Mantel-Haenszel odds ratio; CI: confidence interval

Figure A7.1 Artemisinin derivatives administered in combination compared with monotherapy alone: total failures by day 28 (re-infections included); data from the International Artemisinin Study Group individual patient data meta-analysis *(1)*

Review: Artesunate combination treatments for malaria
Comparison: 01 Artesunate combinations versus no artesunate
Outcome: 02 Parasitological failure by day 28 (failure excludes re-infection)

Study or sub-category	Artesunate n/N	Placebo n/N	OR (fixed) 95% CI	OR (fixed) 95% CI	Quality
02 Background drug: amodiaquine					
Gabon	9/94	21/98		0.39 [0.17, 0.90]	D
Ken_AMRF	35/179	84/182		0.28 [0.18, 0.45]	D
Senegal	16/149	16/141		0.94 [0.45, 1.96]	D
Subtotal (95% CI)	422	421		0.40 [0.28, 0.57]	
Total events: 60 (Artesunate), 121 (Placebo)					
Test for hetetogeneity: Chi² = 7.25, df = 2 (P = 0.03), I² = 72.4%					
Test for overall effect: Z = 5.11 (P < 0.00001)					
03 Background drug: sulfadoxine-pyrimethamine					
Gambia	5/187	17/191		0.28 [0.10, 0.78]	D
Ken_KMRI	37/179	77/181		0.35 [0.22, 0.56]	D
Malawi	18/120	77/113		0.08 [0.04, 0.16]	D
Uganda	24/110	77/131		0.24 [0.13, 0.42]	D
Subtotal (95% CI)	596	616		0.22 [0.17, 2.30]	
Total events: 84 (Artesunate), 242 (Placebo)					
Test for hetetogeneity: Chi² = 13.23, df = 3 (P = 0.004), I² = 77.3%					
Test for overall effect: Z = 9.95 (P < 0.00001)					
Total (95% CI)	1018	1037		0.28 [0.23, 0.35]	
Total events: 144 (Artesunate), 363 (Placebo)					
Test for hetetogeneity: Chi² = 26.35, df = 6 (P = 0.0002), I² = 77.2%					
Test for overall effect: Z = 10.99 (P < 0.00001)					

```
0.001  0.01  0.1    1    10  100 1000
   Favours artesunate      Favours placebo
```

df, degrees of freedom; OR: Mantel-Haenszel odds ratio; CI: confidence interval

Figure A7.2 Artemisinin derivatives administered in combination compared with monotherapy alone: total failures by day 28 (reinfections excluded); data from the International Artemisinin Study Group individual patient data meta-analysis *(16)*

A7.2 Are there any non-artemisinin combination therapies that provide an alternative to standard monotherapy?

A7.2.1 Sulfadoxine-pyrimethamine + chloroquine compared with sulfadoxine-pyrimethamine

Benefits

One systematic review *(2)* (search date 2001), which identified no randomized controlled trials (RCTs) meeting the criteria of at least a 28-day follow-up period for a clinical trial. No subsequent RCTs meeting the inclusion criteria but five with follow-up periods shorter than 28 days *(3–7)*, which are described below.

The first subsequent RCT (160 children and adults, Colombia, 1999-2002), found a lower treatment failure rate at day 21 with the combination treatment than with sulfadoxine-pyrimethamine alone (11/64 (17%) with the combination, 19/79 (26%) with sulfadoxine-pyrimethamine alone, no statistical data reported) *(3)*.

The second subsequent RCT (71 children, Uganda, 2001) found a lower treatment failure rate at day 14 with the combination treatment than with sulfadoxine-pyrimethamine alone (4/32 (13%) with the combination, 5/30 (17%) with sulfadoxine-pyrimethamine alone, no statistical data reported) *(4)*.

The third subsequent RCT (52 children and adults, Lao People's Democratic Republic, 2001) found no significant difference in adequate clinical and parasitological responses at day 14 (20/24 with the combination, 23/28 with sulfadoxine-pyrimethamine alone; relative risk (RR): 1.01, 95% CI: 0.8–1.3) *(5)*.

The fourth subsequent RCT (88 children and adults, Uganda, 2001) found no significant difference in adequate clinical response (27/27 with the combination, 29/29 with sulfadoxine-pyrimethamine alone) *(6)*.

The fifth subsequent RCT (305 children and adults, Uganda, 2001–2002) found no significant difference in adequate clinical response (141/152 with the combination, 119/140 with sulfadoxine-pyrimethamine alone) *(7)*.

Harms

Only one RCT reported on adverse events *(7)*. It found that overall, the incidence of possible adverse events was higher in those receiving the combination therapy than in those receiving sulfadoxine-pyrimethamine monotherapy. This could be explained by the higher incidences of pruritus, nausea and vomiting in the combination group. When mild adverse events were excluded from the analysis, there was no significant difference between the groups. One severe adverse event was reported in the monotherapy group, namely an elevated alanine aminotransferase measurement on day 14 in a girl of 3 years of age. This event was not accompanied by symptoms and resolved within two weeks without medical intervention.

Comment

The systematic review *(2)* identified two RCTs comparing sulfadoxine-pyrimethamine + chloroquine to sulfadoxine-pyrimethamine alone *(8, 9)*. However, neither trial met the WHO inclusion criteria.

The first RCT (85 children aged < 12 years, Papua New Guinea, 1980) compared combination treatment using sulfadoxine-pyrimethamine + an atypical single dose of chloroquine of 10 mg/kg daily to sulfadoxine-pyrimethamine alone *(8)*.

The second RCT (405 children aged 1–10 years, The Gambia, 1995) had a high rate of loss to follow-up (30% in the sulfadoxine-pyrimethamine + chloroquine group, 26% in the monotherapy group) *(9)*.

A7.2.2   Sulfadoxine-pyrimethamine + amodiaquine compared with sulfadoxine-pyrimethamine

Benefits

One systematic review *(2)* (search date 2001), which identified four RCTs, three in Africa *(10–12)* and one in China *(13)* (484 people). One subsequent RCT *(14)*.

Three of the RCTs identified by the systematic review found slightly higher cure rates at day 28 with sulfadoxine-pyrimethamine + amodiaquine than with sulfadoxine-pyrimethamine alone, although the overall difference did not reach statistical significance *(2)*. Similarly, two RCTs (one in Mozambique, and one in China, 1985–1986, 116 people) identified by the review found no significant difference in mean parasite clearance times between the two treatment groups *(10, 13)*. However, the Chinese trial (69 people) found a significantly shorter mean fever clearance time with the combination treatment than with the monotherapy *(13)*.

The subsequent RCT (191 children aged under 10 years, Cameroon, 2001) found a significantly higher adequate clinical response with a negative smear at day 28 with the combination treatment than with the monotherapy *(14)*. Similarly, mean fever clearance time was significantly lower with the combination treatment than with the monotherapy.

Harms

The Chinese trial identified by the systematic review found no significant difference in the rate of adverse events between the two treatment groups (41.7% with the combination, 42.9% with the monotherapy); p value and absolute numbers not reported) *(13)*. Sinus bradycardia and vomiting were the most frequent adverse events overall, and were also more frequent with the combination treatment than with sulfadoxine-pyrimethamine alone (no statistical data reported). However, abdominal pain, headache and dizziness were more common with the monotherapy (no statistical data reported). The Ugandan trial reported no serious adverse effects in either treatment group, whereas that conducted in Mozambique gave no information on adverse events *(10, 11)*. The latter trial (400 people) measured haemoglobin and white blood cell count throughout the follow-up period and found no significant difference between the treatments *(11)*.

The subsequent RCT found a significantly higher rate of fatigue, the most common adverse effect overall, with the combination treatment than with the monotherapy (59/62 (95%) with the combination, 47/62 (76%) with the monotherapy, $p < 0.05$). Similarly, there were higher rates of headache and vomiting with the combination treatment than with the monotherapy (headache: 4/62 (6%) with the combination, 0/62 (0%) with the monotherapy, $p < 0.05$; vomiting: 14/62 (23%) with the combination, 5/62 (8%) with the monotherapy, $p < 0.05$). There was also an increased rate of pruritus with the combination treatment than with sulfadoxine-pyrimethamine alone, although the difference did not reach statistical significance (9/62 (15%) with the combination, 3/62 (5%) with the monotherapy, p value not reported). One person receiving sulfadoxine-pyrimethamine monotherapy presented with purulent vesicles in the thoracic region (no further information provided) *(14)*.

A7.2.3   Sulfadoxine-pyrimethamine + amodiaquine compared with amodiaquine

Benefits

One systematic review *(2)* (search date 2001), which identified three RCTs, one each in China, Mozambique and Uganda) *(10, 11, 13)*. Three subsequent RCTs *(14–16)*.

Two RCTs (150 people in China, 1985–1986 *(13)* and Mozambique, 1986 *(10)* identified by the review found higher parasitological cure rates at day 28 with the combination treatment than with amodiaquine alone. Owing to the apparent heterogeneity between individual study results, the combined relative risk as assessed by several methods did not reach significance (see comment below). These trials found a slightly shorter mean parasite clearance time with the combination treatment than with the monotherapy, although the difference did not reach significance. Similarly, the Chinese trial (97 people) found a shorter mean fever clearance time with the combination treatment than with the monotherapy, although the difference did not reach statistical significance *(13)*. The Ugandan trial *(11)* only reported parasite outcomes at day 7.

The first subsequent RCT (159 children aged 0.5–10.0 years, Nigeria, 2000-2001) found no significant difference in cure rates at day 28 or in mean fever clearance times between the two treatment groups. However, mean parasite clearance time was significantly shorter with the combination treatment than with amodiaquine alone *(15)*.

The second subsequent RCT (127 children aged under 10 years, Cameroon, 2001) found a significantly higher adequate clinical response with negative smear at day 28 with the combination treatment than with amodiaquine alone. However, there was no significant difference in mean fever clearance time between the two groups *(14)*.

The third subsequent RCT (235 children aged 6–59 months, Uganda, 2001) found a lower parasitological failure rate at day 28 with combination treatment *(16)*.

Harms

The Chinese RCT identified by the review reported a slightly higher rate of adverse events with the combination treatment than with amodiaquine alone (41.7% with the combination, 36% with the monotherapy, *p* value not reported) *(13)*. Sinus bradycardia and vomiting were the most frequent adverse events overall and were also more frequent with the combination treatment than with the monotherapy (no statistical data reported). The Ugandan RCT reported no serious adverse effects in either treatment group, whereas that conducted in Mozambique gave no information on adverse events *(10, 11)*.

The first subsequent RCT found three children with sleep disturbance secondary to pruritus but there was no significant difference between the treatments (2/75 with the combination, 1/82 with the monotherapy, *p* value not reported). All other adverse reactions were reported as mild *(15)*.

The second subsequent RCT found no significant difference in fatigue between treatments (59/62 (95%) with the combination treatment, 54/61 (89%) with amodiaquine alone, *p* value not reported). Cutaneous reactions (dermatitis in the hip area in one person and diffuse urticaria at day 5 in one person) were recorded in two people receiving the monotherapy (0/62 (0%) with the combination, 2/61 (3%) with the monotherapy, *p* value not reported) *(14)*.

The third subsequent RCT reported both treatments to be well tolerated and found no serious adverse effects *(16)*.

Comment

The systematic review showed significant differences in parasitological cure rates at day 28 between the two RCTs *(10, 13)*. However, the reviewers found no significant difference between treatments when using a random effects model, or worst and best case scenarios assuming that people lost to follow-up were either all treatment failures or successes *(2)*.

A7.3. How do artemisinin combination therapies compare with non-artemisinin combinations?

A7.3.1 Artesunate + sulfadoxine-pyrimethamine

Benefits

No systematic review. One RCT (276 children aged 6–59 months, Uganda, 2001) comparing artesunate (3 days) + sulfadoxine-pyrimethamine with amodiaquine + sulfadoxine-pyrimethamine *(16)*. It found that parasitological failure at day 28 was significantly increased in the group receiving artesunate (3 days) + sulfadoxine-pyrimethamine compared to that in the group receiving amodiaquine + sulfadoxine-pyrimethamine (PCR-unadjusted treatment failure at day 28: 42/144 (29%) with artesunate (3 days) + sulfadoxine-pyrimethamine, 22/132 (17%) with amodiaquine + sulfadoxine-pyrimethamine; OR: 0.49; 95% CI: 0.27–0.87). However, it found no significant difference in treatment failure rates at day 28 between the two groups once new infections had been excluded (PCR-adjusted treatment failure at day 28: 17/132 (13%) with artesunate (3 days) + sulfadoxine-pyrimethamine, 29/134 (22%) with amodiaquine + sulfadoxine-pyrimethamine; OR: 0.59; 95% CI: 0.29–1.18, $p = 0.14$).

Harms

The same RCT gave no information on adverse events *(16)*.

A7.4 Which is the best artemisinin combination therapy?

A7.4.1 Artemether-lumefantrine (6 doses) compared with artemether-lumefantrine (4 doses)

Benefits

One RCT *(17)*; the RCT (238 adults and children, Thailand, 1996–1997) found a significantly higher rate of cure at day 28 with the 6-dose regimen given over 3 days than with the 4-dose regimen also given over 3 days (PCR-unadjusted treatment cure rate for intention to treat population at day 28: 96/118 (81%); 95% CI: 73.1–87.9% with the 6-dose regimen, 85/120 (71%); 95% CI: 61.8–78.8% with the 4-dose regimen, $p < 0.001$; PCR-adjusted treatment cure rate for evaluable population: 93/96 (97%); 95% CI: 91.1–99.4% with the 6-dose regimen, 85/102 (83%); 95% CI: 74.7–90.0% with the 4-dose regimen, $p < 0.001$).

Harms

The RCT reported all adverse events to be mild or moderate in severity and possibly attributable to malaria *(17)*. It found no adverse cardiovascular effects. It found four serious adverse events that the authors did not consider to be related to treatment. The trial found no changes in QRS duration and PR interval during treatment in 66 people who had regular electrocardiographic monitoring. Similarly, it found no differences in mean and median QTc values between treatment groups.

A7.4.2 Artemether–lumefantrine (6 doses) compared with artesunate (3 days) + mefloquine

Benefits

One systematic review (search date 2004, two RCTs, 419 people, Thailand, 1997–1998 and 1998–1999) *(18)*.

The review found a higher proportion of people with parasitaemia at day 28 with artemether-lumefantrine treatment than with artesunate-mefloquine although the pooled difference did not reach statistical significance (PCR-unadjusted parasitaemia rate 11/289 (4%) with artemether-lumefantrine, 0/100 (0%) with artesunate-mefloquine, RR: 4.20; 95% CI: 0.55–31.93, *p* = 0.2; PCR-adjusted parasitaemia rate 9/289 (3%) with artemether-lumefantrine, 0/100 (0%) with artesunate-mefloquine, RR: 3.50; 95% CI: 0.45–27.03, *p* = 0.2; see comment below). The first RCT (219 adults and children aged over 12 years, Thailand, 1998–1999) identified by the review found no significant difference in median parasite clearance time between the two treatment groups (29 h; 95% CI: 29–32 h in 164 people receiving artemether-lumefantrine, 31 h; 95% CI: 26–31 h in 55 people receiving artesunate-mefloquine, *p* value not reported) *(19)*. Similarly, it found no significant difference in median fever clearance time (29 h; 95% CI: 23–37 h in 76 people receiving artemether-lumefantrine, 23 h; 95% CI: 15–30 h in 29 people receiving artesunate-mefloquine, *p* value not reported) or in median gametocyte clearance time between treatments (72 h; 95% CI: 34–163 h in 26 people receiving artemether-lumefantrine, 85 h; 95% CI: 46–160 h in 10 people receiving artesunate-mefloquine, *p* value not reported). The systematic review did not report results for any other outcomes from the second RCT.

Harms

The systematic review found fewer mild to moderate adverse events with artemether-lumefantrine than with artesunate-mefloquine, although the differences did not reach statistical significance (nausea 4/150 (3%) with artemether-lumefantrine, 6/50 (12%) with artesunate-mefloquine; vomiting 4/150 (3%) compared to 5/50 (10%); sleep disorders: 2/150 (1%) compared to 8/50 (16%); dizziness: 8/150 (5%) compared to 18/50 (36%); *p* values not reported) *(18)*. It found no significant difference in the proportion of people with severe adverse events between the two treatment groups (one person with each treatment).

A7.4.3 Artemether-lumefantrine (6 doses) compared with artesunate (3 days) + amodiaquine

Benefits

No RCTs with a 28-day follow-up period but one (295 children under 5 years of age, Burundi, 2001–2002) with a 14-day follow-up period *(20)*. The trial found no significant difference in the proportion of people with adequate clinical and parasitological response at day 14 between the treatments (140/141 (99.3%); 95% CI: 97.9–100.0% with artemether-lumefantrine, 142/149 (95.3%); 95% CI: 91.9–98.7% with artesunate-amodiaquine, *p* value not reported).

Harms

The RCT found no significant difference in adverse events between the treatment groups other than vomiting, which was significantly less frequent on days 1 and 2 with artemether-lumefantrine than with artesunate-amodiaquine (day 1, 5% with artemether-lumefantrine, 13% with artesunate-amodiaquine; day 2, 1% compared to 5%; *p* values not reported *(20)*.

A7.5 References

1. Adjuik M et al. Artesunate combinations for treatment of malaria: meta-analysis. *Lancet*, 2004, 363:9–17 (search date 2003; primary sources, studies sponsored by the WHO/UNICEF/UNDP/World Bank Special Programme for Research and Training in Tropical Diseases, Medline, Cochrane Controlled Trials Register, and contact with investigators of published trials).

2. McIntosh HM. Chloroquine or amodiaquine combined with sulfadoxine-pyrimethamine for treating uncomplicated malaria. In: *The Cochrane Library, Issue 4*. Chichester, John Wiley & Sons, 2004. (Search date 2001. Primary sources: The Cochrane Infectious Diseases Group trials register, the Cochrane Controlled Trials Register, Medline, Embase, Science Citation Index, African Index Medicus and Lilacs, plus contact with experts in the field and pharmaceutical manufacturers).

3. Blair S et al. Eficacia terapeutica de tres esquemas de traitamiento de malaria no complicado por *Plasmodium falciparum*, Antioquia, Colombia, 2002. [Therapeutic efficacy of 3 treatment protocols for non-complicated *Plasmodium falciparum* malaria, Antioquia, Colombia, 2002.] *Biomedica*, 2003, 23:318–327

4. Ogwang S et al. Clinical and parasitological response of *Plasmodium falciparum* to chloroquine and sulfadoxine-pyrimethamine in rural Uganda. *Wienerische Klinische Wochenschrift*, 2003, 115(Suppl. 3):45–49.

5. Schwobel B et al. Therapeutic efficacy of chloroquine plus sulpha-doxine/pyrimethamine compared with monotherapy with either chloroquine or sulphadoxine/pyrimethamine in uncomplicated *Plasmodium falciparum* malaria in Laos. *Tropical Medicine and International Health*, 2003, 8:19–24.

6. Ndyomugyenyi R, Magnussen P, Clarke S. The efficacy of chloroquine, sulfadoxine-pyrimethamine and a combination of both for the treatment of uncomplicated *Plasmodium falciparum* malaria in an area of low transmission in western Uganda. *Tropical Medicine and International Health*, 2004, 9:47–52.

7. Gasasira AF et al. Comparative efficacy of aminoquinoline-antifolate combinations for the treatment of uncomplicated falciparum malaria in Kampala, Uganda. *American Journal of Tropical Medicine and Hygiene*, 2003, 68:127–132.

8. Darlow B et al. Sulfadoxine-pyrimethamine for the treatment of acute malaria in children in Papua New Guinea. I. *Plasmodium falciparum. American Journal of Tropical Medicine and Hygiene*, 1982, 31:1–9.

9. Bojang KA et al. A trial of Fansidar plus chloroquine or Fansidar alone for the treatment of uncomplicated malaria in Gambian children. *Transactions of the Royal Society of Tropical Medicine and Hygiene*, 1998, 92:73–76.

10. Schapira A, Schwalbach JF. Evaluation of four therapeutic regimens for falciparum malaria in Mozambique, 1986. *Bulletin of the World Health Organization*, 1988, 66:219–226.

11. Staedke SG et al. Amodiaquine, sulfadoxine-pyrimethamine, and combination therapy for treatment of uncomplicated malaria in Kampala, Uganda: a randomised trial. *Lancet*, 2001, 358:368–374.

12. Dinis DV, Schapira A. Étude comparative de la sulfadoxine-pyrimethamine et de l'amodiaquine+sulfadoxine–pyrimethamine dans le traitement du paludisme à Plasmodium falciparum chloroquino-résistant à Maputo, Mozambique [Comparative study of sulfadoxine-pyrimethamine and amodiaquine + sulfadoxine-pyrimethamine for the treatment of malaria caused by chloroquine-resistant Plasmodium falciparum in Maputo, Mozambique.] *Bulletin de la Societéé de Pathologie Exotique,* 1990, 83:521–528.

13. Huang QL et al. [Efficacy of amodiaquine, Fansidar and their combination in the treatment of chloroquine resistant falciparum malaria.] *Zhongguo Ji Sheng Chong Xue Yu Ji Sheng Chong Bing Za Zhi*, 1988, 6:292–295 (in Chinese).

14. Basco LK et al. Therapeutic efficacy of sulfadoxine-pyrimethamine, amodiaquine and the sulfadoxine-pyrimethamine-amodiaquine combination against uncomplicated *Plasmodium falciparum* malaria in young children in Cameroon. *Bulletin of the World Health Organization*, 2002, 80:538–545.

15. Sowunmi A. A randomized comparison of chloroquine, amodiaquine and their combination with pyrimethamine-sulfadoxine in the treatment of acute, uncomplicated, *Plasmodium falciparum* malaria in children. *Annals of Tropical Medicine and Parasitology*, 2002, 96:227–238.

16. Rwagacondo CE et al. Efficacy of amodiaquine alone and combined with sulfadoxine-pyrimethamine and of sulfadoxine pyrimethamine combined with artesunate. *American Journal of Tropical Medicine and Hygiene*, 2003, 68:743–747.

17. van Vugt MV et al. Efficacy of six doses of artemether-lumefantrine (benflumetol) in multidrug-resistant *Plasmodium falciparum* malaria. *American Journal of Tropical Medicine and Hygiene*, 1999, 60:936–942.

18. Omari AA, Gamble C, Garner P. Artemether-lumefantrine for treating uncomplicated falciparum malaria. In: *The Cochrane Library, Issue 4, 2004*. Chichester, John Wiley & Sons (search date 2004, primary sources Cochrane Infectious Diseases Group trials register, the Cochrane Controlled Trials Register, Medline, Embase, Science Citation Index, African Index Medicus and Lilacs, plus contact with experts in the field and pharmaceutical manufacturers).

19. Lefevre G et al. A clinical and pharmacokinetic trial of six doses of artemether-lumefantrine for multidrug-resistant *Plasmodium falciparum* malaria in Thailand. *American Journal of Tropical Medicine and Hygiene*, 2001, 64:247–256.

20. Ndayiragije A et al. Efficacité de combinaisons thérapeutiques avec les dérivés de l'artémisinine dans le traitement de l'accès palustre non-compliqué au Burundi. [Efficacy of therapeutic combinations with artemisinin derivatives in the treatment of non complicated malaria in Burundi.] *Tropical Medicine and International Health*, 2004, 9:673–679.

Annex 8.   Malaria treatment and HIV/AIDS

ANNEX 8

MALARIA TREATMENT AND HIV/AIDS

Malaria and HIV/AIDS share determinants of vulnerability. Given the wide geographical overlap in occurrence and the resulting prevalence of co-infection, the interaction between the two diseases clearly has major public health implications (1). In sub-Saharan Africa, around 300 million cases of malaria occur annually and an estimated 25 million adults and children are living with HIV/AIDS. In 2003 in Africa, HIV/AIDS claimed the lives of an estimated 2.2 million people (2), and malaria 1 million, especially children (3). In South-East Asia, Latin America and the Caribbean there is also significant overlap of these two diseases.

A8.1 Epidemiological overlaps between malaria and HIV/AIDS

The impact of the interaction of malaria and HIV/AIDS is most apparent in areas with generalized HIV/AIDS epidemics and stable malaria. Sub-Saharan Africa carries a high burden of both diseases, thus co-infection is common in many areas. In the most severely affected countries (Central African Republic, Malawi, Mozambique, Zambia and Zimbabwe), more than 90% of the population are exposed to malaria and the prevalence of HIV infection in adults is over 10% (2). In contrast, southern Africa, which has a relatively low burden of malaria, is the worst affected subregion for HIV infection with prevalence as high as 30%. The frequent malaria epidemics in southern Africa may, however, increase the risk of dual infection.

In Latin America and the Caribbean, some overlap of malaria and HIV/AIDS occurs in the general population in Belize, Brazil, El Salvador, Guatemala, Guyana and Honduras. South-East Asian countries, such as Cambodia, Myanmar and Thailand, have a generalized HIV/AIDS epidemic but malaria distribution is heterogeneous in this region. Significant overlap is likely to occur in a number of Indian cities with urban malaria and increasing HIV transmission. Considering that an estimated one billion people in South-East Asia are exposed to unstable malaria, it is clear that even a small overlap of malaria and HIV/AIDS in these settings may have a large public health impact.

A8.2 Evidence of interactions between malaria and HIV/AIDS

A8.2.1 Impact of HIV/AIDS on malaria during pregnancy

There is substantial evidence of the effects of interactions between malaria and HIV/AIDS in pregnant women. HIV infection impairs the ability of pregnant women to control a *P. falciparum* infection *(4, 5)*. They are more likely to develop clinical and placental malaria, more often have detectable malaria parasitaemia and have higher malaria parasite densities in peripheral blood *(6, 7)*. Compared to women with either malaria or HIV infection, co-infected pregnant women are at increased risk of anaemia, preterm birth and intrauterine growth retardation *(8, 9)*. As a result, children born to women with dual malaria and HIV infection are at high risk of low birth weight and death during infancy.

The presence of HIV/AIDS may result in a poorer response to treatment with antimalarials and to intermittent preventive treatment for malaria during pregnancy. Furthermore, there is a risk of adverse reactions if SP for the prevention of malaria in pregnant women and cotrimoxazole (a coformulation of trimethoprim and sulfamethoxazole) for prophylaxis against opportunistic infections are taken together, as both are sulfa-containing medicines.

A8.2.2 Impact of HIV/AIDS on malaria in non-pregnant adults

Evidence on interactions between malaria and HIV/AIDS in non-pregnant adults is accumulating. In areas with stable malaria, HIV infection increases the risk of malaria infection and clinical malaria in adults, especially in those with advanced immunosuppression *(10–12)*. In settings with unstable malaria, HIV-infected adults with AIDS are at increased risk of severe malaria and death *(13, 14)*. Antimalarial treatment failure may be more common in HIV-infected adults with low CD4 cell counts than in those not infected with HIV *(15, 16)*.

A8.2.3 Effects of malaria on HIV infection

Acute malaria episodes cause a temporary increase in replication of HIV and hence in plasma viral load *(17)*. However, so far there is no evidence that malaria has a substantial effect on the clinical progression of HIV infection, HIV transmission or response to antiretroviral treatment in areas where malaria and HIV overlap.

A8.2.4   HIV/AIDS and malaria in children

Few studies have examined the interaction of malaria and HIV/AIDS in children *(18, 19)*. However, HIV-infected children with advanced immunosuppression may have more episodes of clinical malaria and higher parasite densities than those whose immune status is less compromised. In areas of unstable malaria, HIV-infected children may be more likely to experience severe disease or coma *(20)*.

A8.2.5   Drug interactions

There are currently no documented clinical or pharmacological interactions between antimalarials and antiretrovirals. However, pharmacokinetic interactions between certain antimalarials and non-nucleoside reverse transcriptase inhibitors and protease inhibitors are theoretically possible and could lead to toxicity. This suggests that patients receiving protease inhibitors (and the non-nucleoside reverse transcriptase inhibitor delavirdine) should avoid halofantrine. Other antimalarials such as artemether-lumefantrine may also have the potential to interact with antiretrovirals.

Medicines used in the management of opportunistic infections in people living with HIV/AIDS may also interact with antimalarials *(21)*. Interactions are possible between cotrimoxazole, which is used for prophylaxis of opportunistic infections, and SP, which is used for intermittent preventive treatment of malaria in pregnant women in some parts of Africa. It is recommended that SP should not be given if co-trimoxazole is being taken daily as this probably provides an equivalent antimalarial effect. While more research is required, emphasis should be placed on close monitoring and pharmacovigilance in the treatment of malaria and HIV/AIDS.

A8.3   Implications for health systems and service delivery

In HIV-infected individuals, the use of a malaria case definition based on fever alone can result in a febrile illness that may be due to a wide range of ordinary, virulent and opportunistic infections being misdiagnosed and treated as malaria *(22, 23)*. This may lead to inappropriate care of HIV-infected adults with severe febrile illnesses due to causes other than malaria. With the use of more costly antimalarials, it has become necessary to give greater emphasis to parasitological diagnosis *(24)*, and this is particularly important in areas of high prevalence of HIV infection.

In areas affected by malaria and HIV/AIDS, integrated health services are crucial for the introduction of new drugs and diagnostic materials, and offer opportunities for joint planning, training and service delivery.

A8.4   Key recommendations

WHO makes the following recommendations (25).

- HIV-infected pregnant women in areas with stable malaria should – depending on the stage of HIV infection – receive either intermittent preventive treatment for malaria with at least three doses of sulfadoxine-pyrimethamine or daily cotrimoxazole prophylaxis for HIV/AIDS opportunistic infections. Malarial illness in HIV-infected pregnant women who are receiving cotrimoxazole prophylaxis should be managed with non-sulfa antimalarials.

- In areas with stable malaria and a high prevalence of HIV infection, use of a fever-based malaria case definition may result in febrile illnesses caused by opportunistic infections being misdiagnosed as malaria, leading to overtreatment of malaria. Confirmatory parasitological testing for malaria should be applied with high priority in patients at risk of HIV/AIDS (in particular in older children and adults). In addition, health providers should offer HIV testing and counselling.

- In countries with generalized HIV/AIDS epidemics, routine monitoring of antimalarial drug efficacy or effectiveness should include assessment of the effect of HIV on antimalarial treatment outcomes.

- Further research should be undertaken to evaluate possible interactions between antimalarials and antiretrovirals, and pharmacovigilance should be introduced to monitor adverse drug reactions for both the new antimalarials and antiretrovirals.

A8.5   References

1. Hay S et al. The global distribution and population at risk of malaria: past, present, and future. *Lancet Infectious Diseases*, 2004, 4:327–336.

2. *UNAIDS 2004 report on the global AIDS epidemic.* Geneva, Joint United Nations Programme on HIV/AIDS, 2004 (UNAIDS. Report on the global HIV/AIDS epidemic. June 2004).

3. Korenromp EL et al. Measurement of trends in childhood malaria mortality in Africa: an assessment of progress towards targets based on verbal autopsy. *Lancet Infectious Diseases*, 2003, 3:349–358.

4. Steketee RW et al. Impairment of a pregnant woman's acquired ability to limit *Plasmodium falciparum* by infection with human immunodeficiency virus type-1. *American Journal of Tropical Medicine and Hygiene*, 1996, 55:42–49.

5. Ter Kuile F et al. The burden of co-infection with human immunodeficiency virus type 1 and malaria in pregnant women in sub-Saharan Africa. *American Journal of Tropical Medicine and Hygiene*, 2004, 71:41–54.

6. van Eijk et al. Human immunodeficiency virus seropositivity and malaria as risk factors for third-trimester anemia in asymptomatic pregnant women in western Kenya. *American Journal of Tropical Medicine and Hygiene*, 2001, 65:623–630.

7. van Eijk AM et al. The effect of dual infection with HIV and malaria on pregnancy outcome in western Kenya. *AIDS*, 2003, 17, 585–594.

8. Bloland PB et al. Maternal HIV infection and infant mortality in Malawi: evidence for increased mortality due to placental malaria infection. *AIDS*, 1995, 9:721–726.

9. Inion I et al. Placental malaria and perinatal transmission of human immuno-deficiency virus type 1. *Journal of Infectious Diseases*, 2003, 188:1675–1678.

10. Leaver RJ, Haile Z, Watters DA. HIV and cerebral malaria. *Transactions of the Royal Society of Tropical Medicine and Hygiene*, 1990, 84:201.

11. Niyongabo T et al. Prognostic indicators in adult cerebral malaria: a study in Burundi, an area of high prevalence of HIV infection. *Acta Tropica*, 1994, 56:299–305.

12. Whitworth J et al. Effect of HIV-1 and increasing immunosuppression on malaria parasitaemia and clinical episodes in adults in rural Uganda: a cohort study. *Lancet*, 2000, 356:1051–1056.

13. Khasnis AA, Karnad DR. Human immunodeficiency virus type 1 infection in patients with severe falciparum malaria in urban India. *Journal of Postgraduate Medicine*, 2003, 49:114–117.

14. Grimwade K et al. HIV infection as a cofactor for severe falciparum malaria in adults living in a region of unstable malaria transmission in South Africa. *AIDS*, 2004, 18:547–554.

15. Colebunders R et al. Incidence of malaria and efficacy of oral quinine in patients recently infected with human immunodeficiency virus in Kinshasa, Zaire. *Journal of Infection*, 1990, 21:167–173.

16. Birku Y et al. Delayed clearance of *Plasmodium falciparum* in patients with human immunodeficiency virus co-infection treated with artemisinin. *Ethiopian Medical Journal*, 2002, 40(Suppl. 1):17–26.

17. James G K et al. Effect of *Plasmodium falciparum* malaria on concentration of HIV-1-RNA in the blood of adults in rural Malawi: a prospective cohort study. *Lancet*, 2005, 365:233–240.

18. Nguyen-Dinh et al. Absence of association between *Plasmodium falciparum* malaria and human immunodeficiency virus infection in children in Kinshasa, Zaire. *Bulletin of the World Health Organization*, 1987, 65:607–613.

19. Taha T et al. Childhood malaria parasitaemia and human immunodeficiency virus infection in Malawi. *Transactions of the Royal Society of Tropical Medicine and Hygiene*, 1994, 88:164–165.

20. Grimwade K et al. Childhood malaria in a region of unstable transmission and high human immunodeficiency virus prevalence. *Pediatric Infectious Disease Journal*, 2003, 22:1057–1063.

21. Lefèvre G et al. Pharmacokinetics and electrocardiographic pharmacodynamics of artemether-lumefantrine (Riamet®®) with concomitant administration of ketoconazole in healthy subjects. *British Journal of Clinical Pharmacology*, 2002, 54:485–492

22. Francesconi P et al. HIV, malaria parasites, and acute febrile episodes in Ugandan adults: a case–control study. *AIDS*, 2001, 15:2445–450.

23. French N et al. Increasing rates of malarial fever with deteriorating immune status in HIV-1-infected Ugandan adults. *AIDS*, 2001, 15:899–906.

24. *The role of laboratory diagnosis to support malaria disease management: focus on the use of RDTs in areas of high transmission deploying ACT treatment.* Geneva, World Health Organization, in press.

25. *Report of a technical consultation: malaria and HIV interactions and their implications for public health policy: Geneva, Switzerland, 23–25 June 2004.* Geneva, World Health Organization, 2004.

ANNEX 9

TREATMENT OF SEVERE *P. FALCIPARUM* MALARIA

A9.1 Is a loading dose of quinine (20 mg/kg) superior to no loading dose?

Summary

One systematic review, and one subsequent randomized controlled trial (RCT) in children found no significant difference in mortality between quinine regimens with a high initial quinine dose and those with no loading dose. However, parasite and fever clearance times were reduced in the former.

Benefits

One systematic review (search date 2002, three RCTs, 92 people) *(1)*. One subsequent RCT *(2)*.

The systematic review found no significant difference in mortality between a group receiving a high initial dose of quinine (20 mg salt/kg or 16 mg base/kg given by the intramuscular (i.m.) route or by i.v. infusion) followed by a standard dose of quinine, and one receiving the standard dose but no loading dose (two RCTs; 2/35 (5.7%) died in the group receiving a high initial dose, 5/37 (13.5%) with no loading dose; RR: 0.43; 95% CI: 0.09–2.15) *(1)*. One of the RCTs (39 children) found no significant difference between the two groups in mean time to recover consciousness (14 h with a high initial dose, 13 h with no loading dose, weighted mean difference (WMD) 1.0 h; 95% CI: –8.8 h to +10.8 h) *(3)*. Parasite clearance and fever clearance times were shorter for the high initial dose group than for the group with no loading dose (parasite clearance time: two RCTs, 67 people, WMD 7.4 h; 95% CI: –13.2 h to –1.6 h; fever clearance time, two RCTs, 68 people, WMD –11.1 h; 95% CI: –20.0 h to –2.2 h). The subsequent RCT (72 children aged 8 months to15 years in Togo, 1999–2000) found no significant difference between the group receiving a high initial dose of i.v. quinine (20 mg salt/kg over 4 h, then 10 mg salt/kg every 12 h) and that receiving no loading dose (15 mg salt/kg every 12 h) in mortality (2/35 (6%) with a high initial dose, 2/37 (5%) with no loading dose, RR: 1.06; 95% CI: 0.16–7.1) *(2)*. It also found no significant difference between the two groups for recovery of consciousness (35.5 h with a high initial dose, 28.6 h with no loading dose, WMD: +6.9 h; 95% CI: –0.6 h to +14.4 h) or time to 100% parasite clearance (48 h compared to 60 h).

Harms

The systematic review found no significant difference between the groups receiving a high initial dose of quinine and no loading dose in rate of hypoglycaemia (two RCTs; 4/35 (11%) hypoglycaemia with a high initial dose, 3/37 (8%) with no loading dose, RR: 1.39; 95% CI: 0.32–6.00) *(1)*. In one RCT (33 people) included in the review, transient partial hearing loss was significantly increased in the group receiving a high initial dose (10/17 (59%) compared to 3/16 (19%), RR: 3.14; 95% CI: 1.05–9.38) *(4)*. In another (39 children), there was no significant difference between the two groups in neurological sequelae (1/18 (6%) with a high initial dose, 2/21 (10%) with no loading dose, RR: 0.58; 95% CI: 0.06–5.91) *(3)*.

A9.2   Is intramuscular quinine as effective as intravenous quinine?

Summary

One RCT in children found no significant difference between i.m. and i.v. quinine in recovery times or death. However, the study may have lacked the power to detect clinically important differences between treatments.

Benefits

No systematic review. One RCT (59 children aged <12 years, Kenya, 1989-1990), which compared i.m. quinine (20 mg salt/kg loading immediately followed by 10 mg salt/kg every 12 h) with standard-dose quinine given by i.v. infusion (10 mg salt/kg every 12 h) in severe falciparum malaria *(3)*. The trial found no significant difference in mortality, mean parasite clearance time or recovery time to drinking or walking, but may have lacked the power to detect a clinically important difference (mortality: 3/20 (15%) deaths with i.m. quinine, 1/18 (5.6%) with i.v. quinine, RR: 2.7; 95% CI: 0.3–23.7; mean parasite clearance time: 57 h compared to 58 h, WMD: –1.0 h; 95% CI: –12.2 h to +10.2 h; mean recovery times to drinking 47 h compared to 32 h, WMD: +15 h; 95% CI: –5.6 h to + 35.6 h; mean recovery times to walking: 98 h compared to 96 h, WMD: +2.0 h; 95% CI: –24.5 h to +28.5 h).

Harms

Neurological sequelae were reported in two children in the i.m. group, and one child in the i.v. group had transient neurological sequelae that were not specified (2/20 (10%) compared to 1/18 (5.6%), RR: 1.8; 95% CI: 0.2–18.2) *(3)*.

A9.3 Is intrarectal quinine as effective as intravenous or intramuscular quinine?

Summary

One systematic review of 8 trials detected no difference in effect on parasites, clinical illness between the rectal group and either i.m or i.v. groups. Some studies however excluded patients with severe malaria.

Benefits

One systematic review (search date 2005, eight RCTs, 1247 people) *(5)*. Five trials compared intrarectal quinine with i.v quinine infusion, while 6 compared with intramuscular quinine. The systematic review found no significant difference between intrarectal with i.v. or i.m. routes for death, parasite clearance by 48 hours and 7 days, parasite clearance time, fever clearance time, coma recovery time, duration of hospitalization, and time to drinking. However trials reporting these outcomes were small, which resulted in large confidence intervals for all the outcomes.

Harms

No reported rectal irritation. Muciod stools, however, were reported in 4 patients receiving rectal quinine. No statistically significant difference between painful swelling at the site of application or pain at the site of application after administration *(5)*.

A9.4 Is intravenous artesunate superior to intravenous quinine?

Summary

One large multi-centre trial from South-East Asia enrolling 1461 patients (including 202 children less than 15 years old) found a significant advantage of artesunate over quinine in mortality (15% vs 22%). There was an absolute reduction in mortality of 34.7% (95% CI: 18.5–47.6%; $P = 0.002$) in the artesunate group. Quinine was associated with hypoglycaemia (RR: 3.2, $P = 0.009$).

Benefits

No systematic reviews: two RCTs. The first (113 adults with severe malaria, Thailand) comparing i.v. artesunate (2.4 mg/kg initially, 1.2 mg/kg 12 h later, then 1.2 mg/kg daily) to i.v. quinine (20 mg/kg initially, then 10 mg/kg every 8 h) *(6)*. It found no significant difference between the treatments in mortality after 300 h (7/59 (12%) artesunate, 12/54 (22%) quinine, RR: 0.53; 95% CI: 0.23–1.26). It found that artesunate significantly improved parasite clearance time, but that there was no significant difference in fever clearance time or coma recovery time (parasite clearance time: 63 h with artesunate, 76 h with quinine, $p = 0.019$; fever clearance time: 41 h compared to 65 h, $p = 0.2$; coma recovery time: 17 h compared to 18 h, $p = 0.6$).

The second RCT is a large multi-centre trial (SEAQUAMAT study group: Bangladesh, India, Indonesia and Myanmar) with 1431 patients enrolled (7). It found that mortality of 15% (107/730 in the artesunate group was significantly lower than the 22% (164/731) in the quinine group. An absolute reduction of 34.7% (95% CI: 18.5–47.6%; $P = 0.0002$) in the artesunate group. There are, however, still insufficient data for children, particularly from high transmission settings.

Harms

The first RCT found that artesunate significantly reduced hypoglycaemia compared with quinine (6/59 (10%) compared to 15/54 (28%), RR: 0.37; 95% CI: 0.15–0.88) (6). One person treated with artesunate developed an urticarial rash. A similar finding was obtained in the second RCT where treatment with artesunate was well tolerated, whereas quinine was associated with hypo-glycaemia (RR: 3.2; 95% CI: 1.3–7.8; $P = 0.009$) (7).

A9.5   Is intramuscular artemether as effective as intravenous quinine?

Summary

Two systematic reviews and three subsequent RCTs found no significant difference in death rates between the groups receiving artemether and quinine for severe malaria.

Benefits

Two systematic reviews (8, 9) and three subsequent RCTs (10–12). The first review (search date not reported, seven RCTs, 1919 adults and children) analysed individual participant data (8). It found no significant difference in mortality between i.m. artemether and quinine given by i.v. infusion or i.m injection (the latter in one RCT only) in severe falciparum malaria (mortality 136/961 (14%) with artemether, 164/958 (17%) with quinine; OR: 0.80; 95% CI: 0.62–1.02). Parasite clearance was faster with artemether than with quinine (OR: 0.62; 95% CI: 0.56–0.69). The review found no significant difference in the speed of coma recovery, fever clearance time or neurological sequelae between artemether and quinine (coma recovery time, OR: 1.09; 95% CI: 0.97–1.22; fever clearance time, OR: 1.01; 95% CI: 0.90–1.15; neurological sequelae, OR: 0.82; 95% CI: 0.59–1.15).

The second review (search date 1999, 11 RCTs, 2142 people) found a small significant reduction in mortality for i.m. artemether compared with i.v. quinine (OR: 0.72; 95% CI: 0.57–0.91) *(9)*. However, more rigorous analysis excluding three poorer quality trials found no significant difference in mortality (OR: 0.79; 95% CI: 0.59–1.05). The review found no significant difference in neurological sequelae at recovery between the artemether and quinine groups (OR: 0.8; 95% CI: 0.52–1.25).

The first subsequent RCT (105 people aged 15–40 years with cerebral malaria in Bangladesh) compared i.m. artemether (160 mg initially, then 80 mg/kg once daily) with i.v. quinine (loading dose 20 mg/kg, then 10 mg/kg every 8 h) *(10)*. It found no significant difference in death rates between the artemether and quinine groups (9/51 (18%) compared to 10/54 (19%), OR: 0.94; 95% CI: 0.35–2.55). Mean fever clearance time and coma recovery time were significantly longer for artemether than for quinine (fever clearance time: 58 h compared to 47 h, WMD: 11.0 h; 95% CI: 1.6–20.4 h; coma recovery time: 74 h compared to 53 h, WMD: 20.8 h; 95% CI: 3.6–38.0 h). There was no significant difference in mean parasite clearance time between artemether and quinine (52 h compared to 61 h, WMD: 8.6 h; 95% CI: 22.5 h to +5.3 h).

The second subsequent RCT (41 children with severe malaria in Sudan, 40 analysed) compared i.m. artemether (3.2 mg/kg loading dose, then 1.6 mg/kg once a day) with i.v. quinine (loading dose 20 mg/kg, then 10 mg/kg every 8 h) *(11)*. It found that artemether significantly increased fever clearance time but found no significant difference between artemether and quinine in time to parasite clearance (mean fever clearance time: 30.5 h with artemether, 18 h with quinine, $p = 0.02$; mean parasite clearance time: 16 h compared to 22.4 h, $p > 0.05$). There were no deaths in the artemether group, one child died with quinine (0/20 (0%) compared to 1/21 (5%), *p* value not reported).

The third subsequent RCT (77 comatose children aged 3 months–15 years with cerebral malaria) compared i.m. artemether (1.6 mg/kg every 12 h) with i.v. quinine (10 mg/kg every 8 h) *(12)*. It found no significant difference in death rates between the artemether and quinine groups (3/38 (8%) compared to 2/39 (5%), *p* value not reported). There was no significant difference between the two groups in mean fever clearance time, coma recovery time and parasite clearance time (fever clearance time 31 h compared to 36 h; coma recovery time: 21 h compared to 26 h; parasite clearance time 36 h compared to 41 h; *p* values not reported for any comparison).

Harms

The two systematic reviews *(8, 9)* and one of the subsequent RCTs *(3)* found no significant difference in neurological sequelae between the artemether and quinine groups (systematic reviews, see the Benefits section; subsequent trial 3/51 (6%) with artemether, 1/54 (2%) with quinine, RR: 3.18; 95% CI: 0.34–29.56). However, in the first review, rates for the combined outcome of death or neurological sequelae were lower for artemether than for quinine (OR: 0.77; 95% CI: 0.62–0.96, *p* = 0.02) *(8)*.

The second subsequent RCT found that one child treated with quinine developed hypoglycaemia (0/20 (0%) with artemether, 1/21 (5%) with quinine, *(11)*. It reported no neurological problems in either treatment group after 28 days of follow-up.

The third subsequent RCT found no significant difference in transient neurological sequelae between the artemether and quinine groups (2/38 (5%) compared to 1/39 (3%), *(12)*.

Comment

The third subsequent randomized controlled trial did not use loading doses of either artemether or quinine at the beginning of treatment *(12)*. There was a fourth subsequent RCT (52 people) *(13)*. However, it was not clear whether participants had severe malaria, and outcomes were poorly reported.

A9.6 Is intramuscular artemotil as effective as intravenous quinine?

Cochrane Review (search date August 2004). Two small trials (*n* = 194) met the inclusion criteria *(14)*. Both trials compared i.m. artemotil with quinine given by i.v. infusion in children with cerebral malaria and reported on similar outcomes. There was no statistically significant difference in the number of deaths (RR: 0.75; 95% CI: 0.43–1.30, *n* = 194, 2 trials), neurological complications (RR: 1.18;, 95% CI: 0.31–4.46, *n* = 58, 1 trial), or other outcomes including time to regain consciousness, parasite clearance time and fever clearance time. The meta-analyses lack the statistical power to detect important differences.

A9.7 Is rectal artemisinin as effective as intravenous quinine?

Summary

One systematic review of small RCTs found no significant difference in mortality between rectal artemisinin and quinine given by i.v. infusion.

Benefits

One systematic review (search date 1999, three RCTs) comparing rectal artemisinin with i.v. quinine in severe malaria (9). Two RCTs were conducted in 1996–1997. Meta-analysis showed lower mortality with artemisinin and quicker coma recovery time, but the difference was not significant (mortality, three RCTs, 9/87 (10%) with artemisinin, 16/98 (16%) with quinine, RR: 0.73; 95% CI: 0.35–1.50; coma recovery, two RCTs, 59 people, WMD: −9.0 h; 95% CI: −19.7 h to +1.7 h). Fever clearance times were not significantly different (no figures provided).

Harms

One RCT in children found that artemisinin significantly reduced the risk of hypoglycaemia compared with quinine (3/30 (10%) with artemisinin, 19/30 (63%) with quinine, RR: 0.16; 95% CI: 0.05–0.48) (15).

A9.8 Pre-referral treatment with rectal artesunate: should rectal artesunate be used in preference to quinine?

Summary

There are no data from trials with sufficient statistical power to assess differences in mortality following treatment with rectal artesunate and quinine in people with moderate or severe malaria. The objective of the trials that have been conducted was to establish the safety and efficacy of rectal artesunate as pre-referral treatment where there is no access to parenteral treatment. Comparisons between rectal artesunate and i.v. artesunate or i.v., i.m. quinine have been carried out to assess parasitological and clinical response in the 12 or 24 hours immediately after treatment (16, 17).

Benefits

Two randomized, open-label Phase II and three randomised open label Phase III studies have been conducted in people with moderately severe malaria, i.e. patients who could not take drugs by mouth but did not have features of severe malaria and its complications (16, 17). Patients in the artesunate group in the Phase III studies were rescued if their parasitaemia did not decline to below 60% of baseline parasitaemia or if they deteriorated clinically and developed features of severe malaria, convulsions or coma within 24 hours of treatment.

Artesunate had a superior effect in all efficacy measures immediately after treatment. In children treated with artesunate, 80/87 (92%) had a parasite density lower than 60% of baseline, compared to 3/22 (14%) of those who received quinine (RR: 0.09; 95% CI: 0.04–0.19, $p < 0.0001$). In adult, parasitaemia at 12 hours was lower than 60% of baseline in 26/27 (96%) in the artesunate group, compared to 3/8 (38%) in the quinine group. (RR: 0.06; 95% CI: 0.01–0.44, $p < 0.001$). The differences were more significant at 24 h. Artesunate and/or dihydroartemisinin were detected in plasma within 12 h in all adults and in 84/87 of the children.

Harms

A single administration of artesunate suppositories at a dose of 10 mg/kg was well tolerated in both children and adults. There was no significant difference in frequency of adverse events (defined as any new symptom, worsening of any existing symptom, sign or abnormal laboratory value) between treatment groups. Other than local reactions at the site of the i.m. quinine injection in three adult patients, the few adverse events that occurred could have been attributable to falciparum malaria or to pre-existing disease.

A9.9   Should dexamethasone be given routinely?

Summary

One systematic review found no significant difference in mortality between dexamethasone and placebo, but gastrointestinal bleeding and seizures were more common with dexamethasone.

Benefits

One systematic review (search date 1999, two RCTs, 143 people with severe cerebral malaria treated with quinine), which compared dexamethasone with placebo over 48 h (18). One RCT was conducted in Indonesia, the other in Thailand. The review found no significant difference in mortality (14/71 (20%) with dexamethasone, 16/72 (25%) with placebo, RR: 0.89; 95% CI: 0.47–1.68). One RCT found a longer mean time between start of treatment and coma resolution with dexamethasone (76.0 h compared to 57.0 h, $p < 0.02$) (18), but the other found no significant difference (83.4 h compared to 80.0 h, WMD: +3.4 h; 95% CI: −31.3 h to +38.1 h) (20).

Harms

The review found that dexamethasone significantly increased gastrointestinal bleeding and seizures compared with placebo (gastrointestinal bleeding 7/71 (10%) with dexamethasone, 0/72 (0%) with placebo, RR: 8.17; 95% CI: 1.05–63.6; seizures 1/71 (15.5%) compared to 3/72 (4%), RR: 3.32; 95% CI: 1.05–10.47) *(18)*.

Comment

No effect of the steroid on mortality was shown, but the trials were small. Its effect on disability was not reported.

A9.10 Is an initial blood transfusion effective for treating malarial anaemia?

Summary

One systematic review found insufficient data to be sure whether routine administration of blood to clinically stable children (no respiratory distress or cardiac failure) with severe anaemia in endemic malarious areas reduces death, or results in higher haematocrit measured at one month. The review found no significant difference between transfusion and no transfusion for the combined outcome of death or severe adverse events. Transmission of hepatitis B or HIV was not reported. No RCTs examining the effects of transfusion in adults with malaria.

Benefits

One systematic review (search date 1999, RCTs, 230 children with malarial anaemia; packed cell volume range 12–17%) *(21)*. The first RCT (116 children, United Republic of Tanzania) compared initial blood transfusion with conservative treatment, and the second (114 children, The Gambia) compared blood transfusion with iron supplements. Both trials excluded children who were clinically unstable with respiratory distress or signs of cardiac failure. Meta-analysis found fewer deaths in the transfused children, but the difference was not significant (1/118 (1%) with transfusion, 3/112 (3%) with control, RR: 0.41; 95% CI: 0.06–2.70). No RCTs examining the effects of transfusion in adults with malaria.

Harms

The systematic review found that coma and convulsions occurred more often after transfusion (8/118 (6.8%) with transfusion, 0/112 (0%) without, RR: 8.6; 95% CI: 1.1 to 66.0) with seven of the eight adverse events occurring in one of the RCTs. Meta-analysis combining deaths and severe adverse events found no significant difference between children who received transfusions and those who did not (8/118 (7%) with transfusion, 3/112 (3%) without transfusion, RR: 2.5; 95% CI: 0.7–9.3). Transmission of hepatitis B or HIV was not reported *(21)*.

Comment

Studies were small and loss to follow-up was greater than 10%; both of these factors are potential sources of bias. In the first RCT, one child in the transfusion group and one child in the conservative treatment group required an additional transfusion after clinical assessment. In the second RCT, 10 children allocated to receive iron supplements later required transfusion when packed cell volume fell below 12% or they showed signs of respiratory distress.

A9.11 Should phenobarbital be given to patients?

Cochrane Review, search date 2004 *(22)*. Three RCTs with a total of 573 participants met the inclusion criteria. All three compared phenobarbital with placebo or no treatment. In the two trials with adequate allocation concealment, death was more common in the anticonvulsant group (RR: 2.0; 95% CI: 1.20–3.33, fixed-effect model). In all three trials, phenobarbital was associated with fewer convulsions than placebo or no treatment (RR: 0.30; 95% CI: 0.19–0.45, fixed-effect model).

A9.12 Hyperparasitaemia in non-immune or semi-immune populations

Background

Since the classic paper by Field and Niven in 1937 *(23)*, patients with high parasite counts have been known to be at increased risk of dying. Working in Peninsular Malaysia they showed that *P. falciparum* parasite counts of > 100 000/µl of blood (2%) were associated with an increased risk of mortality, while patients with counts of >500 000/µl had a more than 50% chance of dying. Following this observation, hyperparasitaemic patients have been considered to be at high risk. They are often classified as having severe malaria and accordingly treated with parenteral antimalarial drugs wherever possible.

Many hyperparasitaemic patients have evidence of vital organ dysfunction but there is a subgroup of individuals in whom no other manifestations of severe disease occur. These patients have symptoms and signs compatible with a diagnosis of uncomplicated malaria in association with a high parasite count.

They usually have a predominance of young ring forms in the peripheral blood smear, which suggests that the sequestered biomass is relatively small compared with the circulating parasite numbers. On the Thai-Burmese border, the mortality of falciparum malaria in patients with counts of parasitized red blood cells <4% was approximately 0.1%, whereas with counts >4% but without vital organ dysfunction, the mortality was 3% *(24)*. In another study in eastern Thailand, 48 hyperparasitaemic patients were inadvertently included in a cohort of 224 patients (mainly adult men) being followed up after receiving mefloquine treatment for uncomplicated disease in order to identify predictors of treatment failure. Young age, low admission haemoglobin, a history of diarrhoea at the start of treatment or soon after, three or more mefloquine treatments within the preceding year and hyperparasitaemia on an admission blood film were all predictors of subsequent treatment failure *(25)*. The study took place at a time when mefloquine resistance was becoming well established. The authors concluded that, in areas of multidrug resistance, the initial parasite load becomes a critical determinant of treatment failure because strains have intermediate susceptibility to drugs. Patients with little or no immunity to malaria (i.e. children) are at increased risk of treatment failure. In a review of the predictors of treatment failure in a large series of patients studied on the western border of Thailand, the relative risk of treatment failure was increased in patients with parasite counts >10 000/µl (RR: 1.36; 95% CI: 1.12–1.66) *(25)*. In Uganda, it was found that pretreatment parasitaemia >100 000/µl was associated with treatment failure in adults (OR for failure: 2.26; 95% CI: 1.30–3.92), but the authors stated that this was due to a strong association with body temperature in a multivariate analysis *(26)*.

Definition

There is no uniformly agreed definition of hyperparasitaemia. Some publications use a parasite count >100 000/µl of blood. Others use a proportion of parasitized red blood cells >4%, >5% or >10%. In areas of high malaria transmission, mortality rates in patients with 4% or 5% parasitaemia are considerably lower than in areas of low transmission because of the influence of host immunity.

Treatment studies

Is parenteral treatment better?

There are very few studies specifically looking at treatment failure as an outcome in hyperparasitaemic patients. A study working with hyperparasitaemic (>4%) patients in a low-transmission setting, compared oral (artesunate for 3 days + mefloquine on day 2) with i.v. therapy (loading-dose quinine regimen for 24 h followed by mefloquine). Patients in the oral therapy group had significantly faster parasite and fever clearance and shorter hospital stays than those in the intravenous therapy group. No patients progressed to severe disease. However, 28-day cure rates for the oral therapy group were poorer than in non-hyperparasitaemic controls receiving the same treatment (70% compared to 96%). It was concluded that patients with hyperparasitaemia in areas of multidrug resistance need a longer course of treatment to deal with the larger parasite biomass *(27)*.

In one study from a high-transmission setting, 84 hyperparasitaemic (>5%) children aged 1–10 years were assigned at random to receive either 5 days of i.m. artemether or a single oral dose of mefloquine. Cure rates assessed at day 14 were similar in the two groups (98% at day 14 for artemether, 100% at day 28 for mefloquine), although parasite clearance was faster in the artemether group. Four patients in the mefloquine group were excluded because of vomiting, but no patients progressed to severe disease. The authors concluded that oral therapy may be given safely to hyperparasitaemic patients in Africa provided that they can tolerate it orally and the parasites are fully sensitive to the drug *(28)*.

Another study from an area of stable transmission showed rapid parasite clearance in all 32 patients with parasitaemias of 5–35% (mean 10.8%) following oral amodiaquine therapy. Follow-up was to day 14 only and there was no comparative treatment arm. The authors concluded that hyperparasitaemic patients can safely be treated with oral therapy if they have no features of severe disease and can be closely monitored in the first 3 days *(29)*. The same conclusion was reached from another cohort study from an area of stable malaria transmission *(30)*.

Is duration of treatment important?

A study of 100 hyperparasitaemic (>4%) adults and children on the Thai-Burmese border compared treatment with oral artesunate given alone for 5 days with artesunate given for 5 days + mefloquine on day 2. Recrudescence (i.e. treatment failure) rates were 36% and 6% respectively. Two further hyperparasitaemic treatment groups were then investigated: 34 patients with recrudescent malaria following treatment with artesunate + mefloquine who then received artesunate for 7 days; and 132 patients from a malaria vaccine study with primary infections who received artesunate for 7 days + mefloquine on day 2. In these two groups, which were non-randomized and not strictly comparable, recrudescence rates were 26% and 7%, respectively. The authors concluded that duration of treatment is important, particularly when using artemisinin derivatives with short half-lives; that the addition of mefloquine improved cure rates; and that it is important that the parasite counts are reduced massively by artesunate before using mefloquine so that selection pressure for resistance to mefloquine can be minimized *(31)*.

Patients with extreme hyperparasitaemia (>20%)

There have been no treatment studies looking at these patients specifically. They are often treated as having severe malaria even if they can take oral treatment. In low-transmission settings this group of patients was excluded from hyperparasitaemia studies because of the risks of clinical deterioration. Current practice for patients with parasitaemia >20% in these settings is to give parenteral artesunate (or parenteral quinine if artesunate is not available), but this approach is not based on evidence (E. Ashley, personal communication). In Nigeria, where there are higher transmission rates, an upper limit to hyperparasitaemia was not used but the patients with extreme hyperpara-sitaemia were not analysed as a separate group, so no data specific to this group are available.

Conclusions and recommendations

Hyperparasitaemia carries an increased risk of mortality in falciparum malaria. The activity of artemisinin derivatives against circulating parasites makes them particularly effective in hyperparasitaemic patients who have no other signs of severity. Treatment failure rates are higher in hyperparasitaemic patients. This is also a potential source of anew drug resistance.

Hyperparasitaemic patients with no signs of severe disease may be treated with oral artemisinin derivatives provided that the following apply:

- Patients must be monitored closely for the first 48 h after initiation of treatment.
- They must tolerate the drug(s) well, i.e. without diarrhoea or vomiting.
- For regimens containing mefloquine, the mefloquine should be given on day 2 when it is better tolerated, with a lower incidence of early vomiting, rather than on day 0.
- If possible, additional oral artemisinin derivative should be given so that the total treatment course is 5–7 days. This has been studied only for arte-sunate + mefloquine (artesunate 4 mg/kg immediately then 2 mg/kg/day for a further 4–6 days + mefloquine 25 mg/kg given as a split dose after the second day). Alternatively, the first dose of artemisinin derivative can be given parenterally or rectally to ensure adequate absorption.

Non-immune patients with parasitaemia >20% should continue to receive parenteral therapy wherever possible, as there is no evidence for or against using oral treatment in this group and the risks are high.

A9.12 References

1. Lesi A, Meremikwu M. High first dose quinine for treating severe malaria. In: *The Cochrane Library, Issue 2, 2003*. (Oxford: Update Software. Search date 2002; primary sources Cochrane Infectious Diseases Group specialised trials register, Cochrane Controlled Trials Register, Medline, Embase, Lilacs, conference proceedings, researchers working in the field, and hand searches of references).

2. Assimadi JK et al. [Intravenous quinine treatment of cerebral malaria in African children: comparison of a loading dose regimen to a regimen without loading dose]. *Archives de Pediatrie*, 2002, 9:587–594 (in French).

3. Pasvol G et al. Quinine treatment of severe falciparum malaria in African children: a randomized comparison of three regimens. *American Journal of Tropical Medicine and Hygiene*, 1991, 45:702–713.

4. Tombe M, Bhatt KM, Obel AOK. Quinine loading dose in severe falciparum malaria at Kenyatta National Hospital, Kenya. *East African Medical Journal*, 1992, 69:670–674.

5. Eisenhut M, Omari AA. Intrarectal quinine for treating *Plasmodium falciparum* malaria. *Cochrane Database Syst Rev,* 2005, 25(1): CD004009

6. Newton PN et al. Randomized comparison of artesunate and quinine in the treatment of severe falciparum malaria. *Clinical Infectious Diseases*, 2003, 37:7–16.

7. South-East Asian Quinine Artesunate Malaria Trial (SEAQUAMAT) group. Artesunate versus quinine for treatment of severe falciparum malaria: a randomized Trial. *Lancet,* 2005, 366:717-725.

8. Artemether Quinine Meta-analysis Study Group. A meta-analysis using individual patient data of trials comparing artemether with quinine in the treatment of severe falciparum malaria. *Transactions of the Royal Society Tropical Medicine and Hygiene*, 2001, 95:637–650. (Search date not reported; primary sources Medline, Cochrane, and discussions with an international panel of malaria clinical investigators).

9. McIntosh HM, Olliaro P. Artemisinin derivatives for treating severe malaria (Cochrane Review). In: *The Cochrane Library, Issue 2, 2001*. (Oxford: Update Software. Search date 1999; primary sources Cochrane Infectious Diseases Group Trials Register, Medline, Bids, Science Citation Index, Embase, African Index Medicus, Lilacs, hand searches of reference lists and conference abstracts, and contact with organizations and researchers in the field and pharmaceutical companies).

10. Faiz A et al. A randomized controlled trial comparing artemether and quinine in the treatment of cerebral malaria in Bangladesh. *Indian Journal of Malariology*, 2001, 38:9–18.

11. Adam I et al. Comparison of intramuscular artemether and intravenous quinine in the treatment of Sudanese children with severe falciparum malaria. *East African Medical Journal*, 2002, 79:621–625.

12. Satti GM, Elhassan SH, Ibrahim SA. The efficacy of artemether versus quinine in the treatment of cerebral malaria. *Journal of the Egyptian Society of Parasitology*, 2002, 32:611–623.

13. Singh NB et al. Artemether vs quinine therapy in *Plasmodium falciparum* malaria in Manipur – a preliminary report. *Journal of Communicable Diseases*, 2001, 33:83–87.

14. Afolabi BB, Okoromah CN. Intramuscular arteether for treating severe malaria. In: *The Cochrane Database of Systematic Reviews 2004, Issue 4*.

15. Birku Y, Makonnen E, Bjorkman A. Comparison of rectal artemisinin with intravenous quinine in the treatment of severe malaria in Ethiopia. *East African Medical Journal*, 1999, 76:154–159.

16. Krishna S et al. Bioavailability and preliminary clinical efficacy of intrarectal artesunate in Ghanaian children with moderate malaria. *Antimicrobial Agents and Chemotherapy*, 2001, 45:509–516.

17. Barnes KI et al. Efficacy of rectal artesunate compared with parenteral quinine in initial treatment of moderately severe malaria in African children and adults: a randomised study. *Lancet*, 2004, 363:1598–1605.

18. Prasad K, Garner P. Steroids for treating cerebral malaria. In: *The Cochrane Library, Issue 2, 2003*. (Oxford: Update Software. Search date 1999; primary sources Trials Register of the Cochrane Infectious Diseases Group and Cochrane Controlled Trials Register.)

19. Warrell DA et al. Dexamethasone proves deleterious in cerebral malaria. A double-blind trial in 100 comatose patients. *New England Journal of Medicine*, 1982, 306:313–319.

20. Hoffman SL et al. High-dose dexamethasone in quinine-treated patients with cerebral malaria: a double-blind, placebo-controlled trial. *Journal of Infectious Diseases*, 1988, 158:325–331.

21. Meremikwu M, Smith HJ. Blood transfusion for treating malarial anaemia (Cochrane Review). In: *The Cochrane Library, Issue 3, 2001*. (Oxford: Update Software. Search date 1999; primary sources Trials Register of the Cochrane Infectious Diseases Group, Embase, African Index Medicus, Lilacs, hand searches of reference lists, and contact with experts.)

22. Meremikwu M, Marson AG. Routine anticonvulsants for treating cerebral malaria. *The Cochrane Database of Systematic Reviews* 2002, Issue 2. (Article No. CD002152. DOI: 10.1002/14651858.CD002152).

23. Field JW, Niven JC. A note on prognosis in relation to parasite counts in acute subtertian malaria. *Transactions of the Royal Society of Tropical Medicine and Hygiene*, 1937, 30:569–574.

24. Fontanet AL, Walker AM. Predictors of treatment failure in multiple drug-resistant falciparum malaria: results from a 42-day follow-up of 224 patients in eastern Thailand. *American Journal of Tropical Medicine and Hygiene*, 1993, 49:465–472.

25. ter Kuile FO et al. Predictors of mefloquine treatment failure: a prospective study of 1590 patients with uncomplicated falciparum malaria. *Transactions of the Royal Society of Tropical Medicine and Hygiene*, 1995, 89:660–664.

26. Dorsey G et al. Predictors of chloroquine treatment failure in children and adults with falciparum malaria in Kampala, Uganda. *American Journal of Tropical Medicine and Hygiene*, 2000, 62:686–692.

27. Luxemburger C et al. Oral artesunate in the treatment of uncomplicated hyperparasitemic falciparum malaria. *American Journal of Tropical Medicine and Hygiene*, 1995, 53:522–525.

28. Sowunmi A, Walker O, Akindele JA. Severe falciparum malaria: survival with oral therapy. *Tropical and Geographical Medicine*, 1992, 44:352–354.

29. Ndounga M, Basco LK. Rapid clearance of *Plasmodium falciparum* hyper-parasitaemia after oral amodiaquine treatment in patients with uncomplicated malaria. *Acta Tropica*, 2003, 88:27–32.

30. Sowunmi A et al. Open comparison of artemether and mefloquine in uncomplicated *Plasmodium falciparum* hyperparasitaemia in children. *Annals of Tropical Paediatrics*, 1996, 16:5–9.

31. Price R et al. Artesunate and mefloquine in the treatment of uncomplicated multidrug-resistant hyperparasitaemic falciparum malaria. *Transactions of the Royal Society of Tropical Medicine and Hygiene*, 1998, 92:207–211.

ANNEX 10

TREATMENT OF *P. VIVAX*, *P. OVALE* AND *P. MALARIAE* INFECTIONS

A10.1 Introduction

P. vivax, the second major human malaria species, constitutes about 41% of malaria cases worldwide *(1, 2)* and is the dominant species of malaria in many areas outside Africa. It is prevalent in the Middle East, Asia, the Western Pacific and Central and South America. It is rarer in Africa and almost absent from West Africa *(2)*. In most areas where *P. vivax* is prevalent, malaria transmission rates are low and, therefore, the affected populations achieve little immunity to this parasite. Consequently, people of all ages, adults and children alike are at risk of acquiring *P. vivax* infections *(2)*. Where both *P. falciparum* and *P. vivax* prevail, the incidence rates of *P. vivax* tend to peak in people of a younger age than those of *P. falciparum (3)*. The other two human malaria parasite species, *P. malariae* and *P. ovale*, are generally much less prevalent worldwide.

Among the four species of *Plasmodium* that affect humans, only *P. vivax* and *P. ovale* have the ability to form hypnozoites, parasite stages in the liver that can result in relapse infections weeks to months after the primary infection. *P. vivax* preferentially invades reticulocytes and this may lead to anaemia. Repeated infections lead to a chronic anaemia that can affect personal well-being, thereby impairing human and economic development in affected populations. The residual malaria burden of *P. vivax* is likely to be underestimated, and is increasing in some regions of the world *(2)*. Appropriate case management of *P. vivax* malaria will help to minimize the global malaria burden.

Although *P. vivax* is known to be benign malaria, it causes a severe and debilitating febrile illness. Vivax malaria can also occasionally result in severe disease with life-threatening end-organ involvement, similar to severe disease in falciparum malaria. Severe vivax malaria manifestations can present with cerebral malaria *(4)*, severe anaemia *(5)*, jaundice *(5)*, acute respiratory distress syndrome *(6)*, splenic rupture *(7)*, acute renal failure *(8–10)*, severe thrombocytopenia *(7, 11)* and pancytopenia *(5)*. The underlying mechanisms of severe manifestations are not well understood, and may be of an inflammatory pathology similar to that seen in falciparum malaria. During pregnancy, infection with *P. vivax*, as with *P. falciparum*, reduces birth weight. In primegravidae, the reduction is approximately two-thirds that associated with *P. falciparum* (110 g compared to 170 g), but the effect does not decline with successive pregnancies, indeed in the one large series in which this was studied, it increased *(12)*. Chronic anaemia, sequestration and pro-inflammatory cytokines in the placenta lead to lower birth weights *(12, 14)*, increasing the risk of low birth weight (<2500 g) and thus the risk of neonatal death.

A10.2 Diagnosis

Diagnosis of vivax malaria is based on microscopy. RDTs based on immuno-chromatographic methods are available for the detection of non-falciparum malaria. However, their sensitivities for detecting parasitaemias of ≤500/µl are low *(15–21)*. The relatively high cost of these tests is a further impediment to their widespread use in endemic areas. Molecular markers for genotyping *P. vivax* parasites are available for the *dhfr* gene, and those for chloroquine resistance are under development.

A10.3 Treatment

The objectives of treatment of vivax malaria are to cure the acute infection and also to clear hypnozoites from the liver to prevent future relapses. This is known as radical cure.

There are relatively few studies on the treatment of *P. vivax*. Only 11% of the 435 published antimalarial drug trials have been on *P. vivax* malaria *(22)*.

A10.3.1 Standard oral regimen

Chloroquine monotherapy (25 mg base/kg bw over 3 days) is recommended as the standard treatment for vivax malaria because the parasite remains sensitive to chloroquine in much of the world. Primaquine (0.25 or 0.5 mg base/kg bw in a single daily dose for 14 days) is used as a supplement to the standard treatment for the purpose of eradicating dormant parasites in the liver and preventing relapses. The optimal dose of primaquine differs in geographical areas depending on the relapsing nature of the infecting strain, and it remains unclear in patients of heavy body weight *(23)*. This combination of chloroquine and primaquine constitutes treatment to achieve radical cure of vivax malaria.

Primaquine also has weak activity against blood stage parasites. The radical cure regimen of vivax malaria with chloroquine and primaquine therefore conforms to the definition of a combination therapy. The combination of any antimalarial against *P. vivax* infections with primaquine has improved cure rates

(24, 28) and is therefore useful in the treatment of chloroquine-resistant *P. vivax* infections.

A10.3.2 Treatment of drug-resistant *P. vivax*

Therapeutic efficacy data available to date indicate that *P. vivax* remains sensitive to chloroquine throughout most of the world *(26, 29–43)*. Indonesia is exceptional in that high therapeutic failure rates ranging from 5% to 84% have been reported on day 28 of follow-up *(25, 26, 44–49)*. There are reports of chloroquine failure as both treatment and prophylaxis against *P. vivax* malaria from several countries and regions where the species is endemic *(50–53)*. Some of these studies did not measure chloroquine drug concentrations, so that it is questionable whether these findings represented strictly defined chloroquine resistance *(34, 38, 39, 41, 43, 54–57)*.

Antimalarials that are effective against *P. falciparum* are generally effective against the other human malarias. The exception to this is sulfadoxine-pyrimethamine to which *P. vivax* is commonly resistant. Owing to the high prevalence of *dhfr* mutations *(pvdhfr)* in *P. vivax*, resistance to sulfadoxine-pyrimethamine develops faster in this parasite than in *P. falciparum*, and resistant *P. vivax* become prevalent in areas where this drug is used for the treatment of falciparum malaria *(37, 58–66)*.

The recommended treatment for chloroquine-resistant *P. vivax* is quinine (10 mg salt/kg bw three times a day for 7 days) *(67)*. However, it is not an ideal treatment because of the toxicity of quinine and the poor adherence to this regimen. A study in Thailand has found that treatment of vivax malaria with quinine leads to early relapses. This may be because quinine has a short half-life, and no antihypnozoite activity *(37)*.

Other treatments that have been tested for the treatment of *P. vivax* malaria with varying degrees of efficacy include the following drugs.

Amodiaquine (25–30 mg base/kg bw given over 3 days) has been used effectively for the treatment of chloroquine-resistant vivax malaria *(67)* and has been well tolerated *(68–70)*. Primaquine must be added for radical cure. Mild nausea, vomiting and abdominal pain are the commonly reported adverse reactions *(70)*.

Mefloquine (15 mg base/kg bw as a single dose) has been found to be highly effective with a treatment success of 100% *(37)*.

Halofantrine (24 mg base/kg bw over 12 hours in three divided doses) has shown varied efficacy in vivax malaria *(24, 25, 36, 37)* but is not recommended because of its known cardiotoxicity.

Doxycycline alone (100 mg twice a day for 7 days) is not recommended for the treatment of vivax malaria because of its poor efficacy *(46)*.

Artemisinin derivatives as monotherapy for 3–7 days have shown poor efficacy in vivax malaria, with day 28 cure rates of 47–77% *(27, 37, 55)*. The addition of primaquine to these regimes improved the day 28 cure rates to 100% *(27, 71)*.

Combinations of chloroquine (25 mg base/kg bw given in divided doses over 3 days) and sulfadoxine-pyrimethamine (based on a pyrimethamine dosage of 1.25 mg/kg bw as a single dose) or chloroquine (25 mg base/kg bw in divided doses over 3 days) and doxycycline (100 mg twice a day for 7 days) have shown modest efficacy (71–82%) and have not shown significant improvements in cure rate compared with chloroquine alone *(46, 70)*.

Other combinations of artesunate (4 mg/kg bw, single daily dose for 3 days) and sulfadoxine-pyrimethamine (based on a pyrimethamine dosage of 1.25 mg/kg bw, single dose), when used in areas of high chloroquine-resistant *P. vivax* (west Papua), produced 28-day cure rates of less than 90% *(64)*.

Artemether-lumefantrine (the latter formerly known as benflumetol) (16 tablets for 3 days or 20 tablets for 5 days given twice a day in divided doses) has shown significantly shorter parasite clearance times than in the standard regimen of chloroquine + primaquine. However, these regimens were associated with higher relapse rates than with chloroquine + primaquine in the nine months of follow up *(72)*. In another evaluation of the efficacy of artemether-lumefantrine against *P. falciparum* the population studied included patients who were also infected with *P. vivax*. Although high rates of *P. vivax* parasite clearance were noted within 42 h, in 6/16 patients parasites reappeared before 28 days *(73)*.

The best combinations for the treatment of *P. vivax* are those containing primaquine when given at antihypnozoite doses *(24, 29, 37, 39, 56, 70, 74, 75)*. The addition of primaquine at the standard dose of 0.25 mg/kg bw, once daily for 14 days to chloroquine has improved the cure rates in chloroquine-resistant vivax malaria *(25, 39, 54, 56)*. Further, at higher doses (0.5–0.6 mg/kg, once daily for 14 days), primaquine appears to be effective in areas where there are presumed primaquine-resistant hypnozoite infections *(27, 76)*.

Unlike *P. falciparum*, *P. vivax* cannot be cultured continuously *in vitro*, so that it is more difficult to determine the *in vitro* sensitivity of *P. vivax* to antimalarials. *In vivo* assessment of the therapeutic efficacy of drugs against *P. vivax* malaria is also compounded by difficulties in distinguishing recrudescences due to drug-resistant infections from relapses. The interval between the primary and repeat infection can serve as a general guide. If the recurrence appears within 16 days of starting treatment of the primary infection it is almost certainly a recrudescence due to therapeutic failure. A recurrence between days 17 and

28 may be either a recrudescence by chloroquine-resistant parasites or a relapse. Beyond day 28 any recurrence probably represents a relapse in an infection of chloroquine-sensitive *P. vivax (77, 78)*. A recurrent vivax parasitaemia in the presence of chloroquine blood levels exceeding 100 ng/ml, and a parasite genotype identical with the primary infection as detected by PCR are more suggestive of chloroquine resistance of the primary infection than a relapse infection.

A10.3.3 Preventive therapy for relapses

Primaquine is the only available and marketed drug that can eliminate the latent hypnozoite reservoirs of *P. vivax* and *P. ovale* that cause relapses. There is no evidence that treatment courses shorter than 14 days are effective in preventing relapses *(39, 56, 79, 80)*. Relapse rates and primaquine sensitivity vary geographically. The reported incidences of relapses range from 11–26.7% in India *(56, 81)* to 49–51% in Afghanistan *(79)*. Relapses may occur one to four times after initiation of radical treatment *(80, 82)*. In patients treated with chloroquine, the first relapse is often suppressed by pharmacologically active concentrations of chloroquine and therefore does not manifest clinically or parasitologically. The first clinically manifested relapse has been reported any time after day 16 and up to four years following the primary infection *(83, 85)*. Host immunity is also considered to be a major contributor to the therapeutic response against relapses *(86)*. Risk factors associated with relapses are female sex, higher parasitaemia at baseline, shorter number of days with symptoms prior to baseline, and a lower dose of primaquine *(83)*.

Hypnozoites of many strains of *P. vivax* are susceptible to a total dose of 210 mg of primaquine *(24, 37, 54, 75, 79, 83, 87)*. Infections with the Chesson strain or primaquine-resistant strains prevalent in southern regions of South-East Asia and Oceania require a higher dosage of primaquine (22.5 mg or 30 mg per day for 14 days for a total dose of 315 mg or 420 mg, respectively) to prevent relapses *(56, 74, 76)*. Primaquine is contraindicated in patients with severe variants of the inherited enzyme deficiency, G6PD *(88, 89)* (see section below on adverse effects).

Although, the long 14-day course of primaquine is a clear disadvantage, it has been shown that poor adherence to unsupervised 14-day primaquine therapy can be overcome effectively through patient education *(90)*. The lengthy treatment courses and follow-up periods make the assessment of primaquine efficacy difficult. Thus, the identification of *P. vivax* strains that are resistant to chloroquine and/or to primaquine presents major challenges.

Alternative drugs are much needed for the radical treatment of *P. vivax* malaria resistant to chloroquine and/or primaquine. A new drug, tafenoquine, is currently being evaluated as an alternative to primaquine in the prevention of relapses *(91)*. However, this too has haemolytic potential in G6PD-deficient individuals.

A10.3.4 Treatment of severe and complicated vivax malaria

Prompt and effective management should be the same as for severe and complicated falciparum malaria (set out in section 8 of the main document).

A10.3.5 Treatment of malaria caused by *P. ovale* and *P. malariae*

Resistance of *P. ovale* and *P. malariae* to antimalarials is not well characterized and these infections are considered to be generally sensitive to chloroquine. Only a single study in Indonesia has reported *P. malariae* resistant to chloroquine *(63)*. The recommended treatment for radical cure of *P. ovale*, another relapsing malaria, is the same as that for *P. vivax,* i.e. with chloroquine and primaquine. The high prevalence of G6PD-deficiency status in areas endemic for *P. ovale* calls for the same caution in the use of primaquine as stated in section A10.3.3. *P. malariae* forms no hypnozoites and so does not require radical cure with primaquine.

A10.3.6 Adverse effects and contraindications

Chloroquine is generally well tolerated. Common adverse effects include mild dizziness, nausea, vomiting, abdominal pain and itching *(3, 67 86)*.

Primaquine can induce a life-threatening haemolysis in those who are deficient in the enzyme G6PD (see section A10.3.3). A full course of primaquine, given as a daily dose of 0.25 mg base/kg bw for 14 days, is reported to be safe in populations where G6PD deficiency is either absent or readily diagnosable but could induce a self-limiting haemolysis in those with mild G6PD deficiency *(34, 54, 56)*. To reduce the risk of haemolysis in such individuals, an intermittent primaquine regimen of 0.75 mg base/kg weekly for 8 weeks can be given under medical supervision. This regimen is safe and effective *(89)*. In non-G6PD deficient individuals, a high dose of primaquine (30 mg/day) has been shown to be safe and effective for Chesson strain *P. vivax* malaria in South-East Asia during a 28-day follow-up *(27, 74, 76)*. In regions where prevalence of G6PD deficiency is relatively high, G6PD testing is required before administration of primaquine. Primaquine is not recommended during pregnancy and in infancy since limited safety data are available in these groups *(67)*. Abdominal pain and/or cramps are commonly reported when primaquine is taken on an empty stomach. Gastrointestinal toxicity is dose-related and is improved by taking primaquine with food. Primaquine may cause weakness, uneasiness in the chest, haemolytic anaemia, methaemoglobinaemia (which occurs in nonhaemolysed red cells), leukopenia, and suppression of myeloid series. Therefore, primaquine should not be given in conditions predisposing to granulocytopenia, including rheumatoid arthritis and lupus erythematosus.

A10.4 Monitoring therapeutic efficacy

There is a need to monitor the antimalarial sensitivity of *P. vivax* in order to improve the treatment of vivax malaria, in particular in view of its emerging resistance to chloroquine. An *in vitro* test system has been developed for assessing the parasite's sensitivity to antimalarials *(92, 93)*. A modified version of the standard WHO *in vitro* microtest for determination of the antimalarial sensitivity of *P. falciparum* has been used successfully for assessing the antimalarial sensitivity of *P. vivax* populations and for screening the efficacy of new antimalarials by measuring minimal inhibitory concentration (MIC), and the concentrations providing 50% and 90% inhibition (IC_{50}), and (IC_{90}) *(87, 89)*. WHO has also recently introduced a revised protocol for *in vivo* monitoring of the therapeutic efficacy of chloroquine in *P. vivax* malaria *(95)*. The revised protocol includes measurement of blood chloroquine levels, PCR genotyping and the use of molecular markers (only available for the *dhfr* gene) to help clarify and complete the overall picture of drug resistance. A better understanding of the molecular mechanisms underlying drug resistance in *P. vivax* is needed to improve the monitoring of chloroquine resistance.

A10.5 Conclusions and recommendations

- The standard oral regimen of chloroquine of 25 mg base/kg bw given over 3 days + primaquine at either a low (0.25 mg base/kg bw per day for 14 days) or high (0.5–0.75 mg base/kg bw per day for 14 days) dose is effective and safe for the radical cure of chloroquine-sensitive *P. vivax* malaria in patients with no G6PD deficiency.

- Of the limited alternative treatments that have been evaluated, amodiaquine is a promising monotherapy and has been shown to be effective for the treatment of chloroquine-resistant *P. vivax* malaria (cure rate >90%).

- In areas where infections of drug-resistant *P. falciparum* and/or *P. vivax* are common, drug regimens to treat both species effectively must be used. An ACT that does not include sulfadoxine-pyrimethamine would be a good choice.

- The use of high-dose primaquine (0.5–0.75 mg base/kg bw per day for 14 days), with either chloroquine or another effective antimalarial, is essential for trying to prevent relapses of primaquine-resistant or primaquine-tolerant *P. vivax*.

- A primaquine regimen of 0.75 mg base/kg bw once per week for 8 weeks is recommended as antirelapse therapy for *P. vivax* and *P. ovale* malaria in patients with mild G6PD deficiency.

- Increased efforts are needed to evaluate alternative treatments for *P. vivax* strains that are resistant to chloroquine. Urgent needs include establishing *in vitro* culture of *P. vivax* to permit the assessment of drug susceptibility, research to improve understanding of the molecular mechanisms of drug resistance, and the development of better tools for genotyping *P. vivax*.

A10.6 References

1. Hay SI et al. The global distribution and population at risk of malaria: past, present, and future. *Lancet Infectious Diseases,* 2004, 4: 327–336.

2. Mendis K et al. The neglected burden of *Plasmodium vivax* malaria. *American Journal of Tropical Medicine and Hygiene,* 2001, 64:97–106.

3. Tjitra E. *Improving the diagnosis and treatment of malaria in Eastern Indonesia* [dissertation]. Menzies School of Health Research, Northern Territory University, Darwin, Australia, 2001.

4. Beg MA et al. Cerebral involvement in benign tertian malaria. *American Journal of Tropical Medicine and Hygiene,* 2002, 67:230–232.

5. Mohapatra MK et al. Atypical manifestations of *Plasmodium vivax* malaria. *Indian Journal of Malariology,* 2002, 39:18–25.

6. Tanios MA et al. Acute respiratory distress syndrome complicating *Plasmodium vivax* malaria. *Critical Care Medicine,* 2001, 29:665–667.

7. Oh MD et al. Clinical features of vivax malaria. *American Journal of Tropical Medicine and Hygiene,* 2001, 65:143–146.

8. Mehta KS et al. Severe acute renal failure in malaria. *Journal of Postgraduate Medicine,* 2001, 47:24–26.

9. Naqvi R et al. Outcome in severe acute renal failure associated with malaria. *Nephrology, Dialysis, Transplantation,* 2003, 18:1820–1823.

10. Prakash J et al. Acute renal failure in *Plasmodium vivax* malaria. *Journal of the Association of Physicians of India,* 2003, 51:265–267.

11. Makkar RP et al. *Plasmodium vivax* malaria presenting with severe thrombocytopenia. *Brazilian Journal of Infectious Diseases,* 2002, 6:263–265.

12. Nosten F et al. Effects of *Plasmodium vivax* malaria in pregnancy. *Lancet,* 1999, 354:546–549.

13. Udomsangpetch R et al. Rosette formation by *Plasmodium vivax. Transactions of the Royal Society of Tropical Medicine and Hygiene*, 1995, 89:635–637.

14. Fried M et al. Malaria elicits type 1 cytokines in the human placenta: IFN-gamma and TNF-alpha associated with pregnancy outcomes. *Journal of Immunology*, 1998, 160:2523–2530.

15. Tjitra E et al. Field evaluation of the ICT malaria P.f/P.v immunochromatographic test for detection of *Plasmodium falciparum* and *Plasmodium vivax* in patients with a presumptive clinical diagnosis of malaria in eastern Indonesia. *Journal of Clinical Microbiology*, 1999, 37:2412–2417.

16. Coleman RE et al. Field evaluation of the ICT Pf/Pv immunochromatographic test for the detection of asymptomatic malaria in a *Plasmodium falciparum/vivax* endemic area in Thailand. *American Journal of Tropical Medicine and Hygiene*, 2002, 66:379–383.

17. Iqbal J, Khalid N, Hira PR. Comparison of two commercial assays with expert microscopy for confirmation of symptomatically diagnosed malaria. *Journal of Clinical Microbiology*, 2002, 40:4675–4678.

18. Farcas GA et al. Evaluation of the Binax NOW ICT test versus polymerase chain reaction and microscopy for the detection of malaria in returned travelers. *American Journal of Tropical Medicine and Hygiene*, 2003, 69:589–592.

19. Figueiredo FAF et al. Performance of an immunochromatography test for vivax malaria in the Amazon region, Brazil. *Revista de Saude Publica*, 2003, 37:390–392.

20. Forney JR et al. Devices for rapid diagnosis of malaria: evaluation of prototype assays that detect *Plasmodium falciparum* histidine-rich protein 2 and a *Plasmodium vivax*-specific antigen. *Journal of Clinical Microbiology*, 2003, 41:2358–2366.

21. Kolaczinski J et al. Comparison of the OptiMAL rapid antigen test with field microscopy for the detection of *Plasmodium vivax* and *P. falciparum*: considerations for the application of the rapid test in Afghanistan. *Annals of Tropical Medicine and Parasitology*, 2004, 98:15–20.

22. Myint HY et al. A systematic overview of published antimalarial drug trials. *Transactions of the Royal Society of Tropical Medicine and Hygiene*, 2004, 98:73–81.

23. Schwartz E, Regev-Yochay G, Kurnik D. Short report: a consideration of primaquine dose adjustment for radical cure of *Plasmodium vivax* malaria. *American Journal of Tropical Medicine and Hygiene*, 2000, 62:393–395.

24. Tjitra E et al. Randomized comparative study of chloroquine and halofantrine in vivax malaria patients. *Medical Journal of Indonesia*, 1995, 4:30–36.

25. Baird JK et al. Treatment of chloroquine-resistant *Plasmodium vivax* with chloroquine and primaquine or halofantrine. *Journal of Infectious Diseases,* 1995, 171:1678–1682.

26. Fryauff DJ et al. Survey of in vivo sensitivity to chloroquine by *Plasmodium falciparum* and *P. vivax* in Lombok, Indonesia. *American Journal of Tropical Medicine and Hygiene,* 1997, 56: 241–244.

27. Silachamroon U et al. Clinical trial of oral artesunate with or without high-dose primaquine for the treatment of vivax malaria in Thailand. *American Journal of Tropical Medicine and Hygiene,* 2003, 69:14–18.

28. Baird JK, Rieckmann KH. Can primaquine therapy for vivax malaria be improved? *Trends in Parasitology,* 2003, 19:115–120.

29. Tan-ariya P et al. Clinical response and susceptibility in vitro of *Plasmodium vivax* to the standard regimen of chloroquine in Thailand. *Transactions of the Royal Society of Tropical Medicine and Hygiene,* 1995, 89:426–429.

30. Baird JK et al. Survey of resistance to chloroquine by *Plasmodium vivax* in Indonesia. *Transactions of the Royal Society of Tropical Medicine and Hygiene,* 1996, 90:409–411.

31. Baird JK et al. Chloroquine sensitive *Plasmodium falciparum* and *P. vivax* in central Java, Indonesia. *Transactions of the Royal Society of Tropical Medicine and Hygiene,* 1996, 90:412–413.

32. Baird JK et al. Survey of resistance to chloroquine of falciparum and vivax malaria in Palawan, The Philippines. *Transactions of the Royal Society of Tropical Medicine and Hygiene,* 1996, 90:413–4144.

33. Fryauff DJ et al. Survey of resistance *in vivo* to chloroquine of *Plasmodium falciparum* and *P. vivax* in North Sulawesi, Indonesia. *Transactions of the Royal Society of Tropical Medicine and Hygiene,* 1998, 92:82–83.

34. Looareesuwan S et al. Chloroquine sensitivity of *Plasmodium vivax* in Thailand. *Annals of Tropical Medicine and Parasitology,* 1999, 93:225–230.

35. Fryauff DJ et al. *In vivo* responses to antimalarials by *Plasmodium falciparum* and *P. vivax* from isolated Gag island of northwest Irian Jaya, Indonesia. *American Journal of Tropical Medicine and Hygiene,* 1999, 60:542–546.

36. Taylor WRJ et al. Assessing drug sensitivity of *Plasmodium vivax* to halofantrine or chloroquine in southern, central Vietnam using an extended 28-day *in vivo* test and polymerase chain reaction genotyping. *American Journal of Tropical Medicine and Hygiene,* 2000, 62:693–697.

37. Pukrittayakamee S et al. Therapeutic responses to different antimalarial drugs in vivax malaria. *Antimicrobial Agents and Chemotherapy,* 2000, 44:1680–1685.

38. McGready R et al. The effects of quinine and chloroquine antimalarial treatments in the first trimester of pregnancy. *Transactions of the Royal Society of Tropical Medicine and Hygiene*, 2002, 96:180–184.

39. Yadav RS, Ghosh SK. Radical curative efficacy of five-day regimen of primaquine for treatment of *Plasmodium vivax* malaria in India. *Journal of Parasitology*, 2002, 88:1042–1044.

40. Nandy A et al. Monitoring the chloroquine sensitivity of *Plasmodium vivax* from Calcutta and Orissa, India. *Annals of Tropical Medicine and Parasitology*, 2003, 97:215–220.

41. Baird JK et al. Chloroquine for the treatment of uncomplicated malaria in Guyana. *Annals of Tropical Medicine and Parasitology*, 2002, 96:339–348.

42. Castillo CM, Osorio LE, Palma GI. Assessment of therapeutic response of *Plasmodium vivax* and *Plasmodium falciparum* to chloroquine in a malaria transmission free area in Colombia. *Memorias do Instituto Oswaldo Cruz*, 2002, 97:559–562.

43. Ruebush TK et al. Chloroquine-resistant *Plasmodium vivax* malaria in Peru. *American Journal of Tropical Medicine and Hygiene*, 2003, 69:548–552.

44. Baird JK et al. *In vivo* resistance to chloroquine by *Plasmodium vivax* and *Plasmodium falciparum* at Nabire, Irian Jaya, Indonesia. *American Journal of Tropical Medicine and Hygiene*, 1997, 56:627–631.

45. Fryauff DJ et al. Chloroquine-resistant *Plasmodium vivax* in transmigration settlements of West Kalimantan, Indonesia. *American Journal of Tropical Medicine and Hygiene*, 1998, 59:513–518.

46. Taylor WRJ et al. Chloroquine/doxycycline combination versus chloroquine alone and doxycycline alone for the treatment of *Plasmodium falciparum* and *Plasmodium vivax* malaria in northeastern Irian Jaya, Indonesia. *American Journal of Tropical Medicine and Hygiene*, 2001, 64:223–228.

47. Fryauff DJ et al. The drug sensitivity and transmission dynamics of human malaria on Nias Island, North Sumatra, Indonesia. *Annals of Tropical Medicine and Parasitology*, 2002, 96:447–462.

48. Maguire JD et al. Chloroquine-resistant *Plasmodium malariae* in south Sumatra, Indonesia. *Lancet*, 2002, 360:58–60.

49. Sumawinata IW et al. Very high risk of therapeutic failure with chloroquine for uncomplicated *Plasmodium falciparum* and *P. vivax* malaria in Indonesian Papua. *American Journal of Tropical Medicine and Hygiene*, 2003, 68:416–420.

50. Schuurkamp GJ et al, Chloroquine-resistant *Plasmodium vivax* in Papua New Guinea. *Transactions of the Royal Society of Tropical Medicine and Hygiene*, 1992, 86:121–122.

51. Myat-Phone-Kyaw et al. Emergence of chloroquine-resistant Plasmodium vivax in Myanmar (Burma). *Transactions of the Royal Society of Tropical Medicine and Hygiene,* 1993, 87:687.

52. Marlar-Than et al. Development of resistance to chloroquine by *Plasmodium vivax* in Myanmar. *Transactions of the Royal Society of Tropical Medicine and Hygiene,* 1995, 89:307–308.

53. Dua VK, Kar PK, Sharma VP. Chloroquine resistant *Plasmodium vivax* malaria in India. *Tropical Medicine and International Health,* 1996, 1:816–819.

54. Buchachart K et al. Effect of primaquine standard dose (15 mg/day for 14 days) in the treatment of vivax malaria patients in Thailand. *Southeast Asian Journal of Tropical Medicine and Public Health,* 2001, 32:720–726.

55. Phan GT et al. Artemisinin or chloroquine for blood stage *Plasmodium vivax* malaria in Vietnam. *Tropical Medicine and International Health,* 2002, 7:858–864.

56. Gogtay NJ et al. Efficacies of 5- and 14-day primaquine regimens in the prevention of relapse in *Plasmodium vivax* infections. *Annals of Tropical Medicine and Parasitology,* 1999, 93:809–812.

57. Alecrim MC, Alecrim W, Macedo V. *Plasmodium vivax* resistance to chloroquine (R2) and mefloquine (R3) in Brazilian Amazon region. *Revista da Sociedade Brasiliera de Medicina Tropical,* 1999, 32:67–68.

58. Young MD, Burgens RW. Pyrimethamine resistance in *Plasmodium vivax* malaria. *Bulletin of the World Health Organization,* 1959, 20:27–36.

59. Laing AB. Hospital and field trials of sulformethoxine with pyrimethamine against Malaysian strains of *Plasmodium falciparum* and *P. vivax*. *Medical Journal of Malaysia,* 1968, 23:5–19.

60. Doberstyn EB et al. Treatment of vivax malaria with sulfadoxine-pyrimethamine and with pyrimethamine alone. *Transactions of the Royal Society of Tropical Medicine and Hygiene,* 1979, 73:15–17.

61. De Pecoulas PE et al. Sequence variations in the *Plasmodium vivax* dihydrofolate reductase-thymidylate synthase gene and their relationship with pyrimethamine resistance. *Molecular Biochemistry and Parasitology,* 1998, 92:265–273.

62. Imwong M et al. Association of genetic mutations in *Plasmodium vivax dhfr* with resistance to sulfadoxine-pyrimethamine geographical and clinical correlates. *Antimicrobial Agents and Chemotherapy,* 2001, 45:3122–3127.

63. Maguire JD et al. Chloroquine or sulfadoxine-pyrimethamine for the treatment of uncomplicated *Plasmodium falciparum* malaria during an epidemic in Central Java, Indonesia. *Annals of Tropical Medicine and Parasitology,* 2002, 96:655–668.

64. Tjitra E et al. Efficacies of artesunate-sulfadoxine-pyrimethamine and chloroquine-sulfadoxine-pyrimethamine in vivax malaria pilot studies: relationship to *Plasmodium vivax dhfr* mutations. *Antimicrobial Agents and Chemotherapy,* 2002, 46:3947–3053.

65. Imwong M et al. Novel point mutations in the dihydrofolate reductase gene of *Plasmodium vivax:* evidence for sequential selection by drug pressure. *Antimicrobial Agents and Chemotherapy,* 2003, 47:1514–1521.

66. Hastings MD et al. Dihydrofolate reductase mutations in *Plasmodium vivax* from Indonesia and therapeutic response to sulfadoxine plus pyrimethamine. *Journal of Infectious Diseases,* 2004, 189:744–750.

67. *The use of antimalarial drugs. Report of an informal consultation.* Geneva, World Health Organization, 2001.

68. Cooper RD, Rieckmann KH. Efficacy of amodiaquine against a chloroquine-resistant strain of *Plasmodium vivax. Transactions of the Royal Society of Tropical Medicine and Hygiene,* 1990, 84: 473.

69. Rieckmann KH. Monitoring the response of malaria infections to treatment. *Bulletin of the World Health Organization,* 1990, 68:759–760.

70. Tjitra E. *Randomised comparative study of the therapeutic efficacy of chloroquine alone versus combined chloroquine plus sulphadoxine-pyrimethamine and amodiaquine alone for the treatment of vivax malaria in Bangka island, Indonesia* (Report of the WHO funded study). 2003, Jakarta, National Institute of Health Research and Development, Ministry of Health, Republic Indonesia.

71. da Silva RS et al. Short course schemes for vivax malaria treatment. *Revista da Sociedade Brasiliera de Medicina Tropical,* 2003, 36:235–239.

72. Li X et al. [Observation on efficacy of artemether compound against vivax malaria.] *Zhongguo Ji Sheng Chong Xue Yu Ji Sheng Chong Bing Za Zhi* [Chinese journal of parasitology and parasitic disease], 1999, 17:175–177 [in Chinese].

73. Lefèvre G et al. A clinical and pharmacokinetic trial of six doses of artemether-lumefantrine for multidrug resistant *Plasmodium falciparum* malaria in Thailand. *American Journal of Tropical Medicine and Hygiene,* 2001, 64:247–256.

74. Fryauff DJ et al. Halofantrine and primaquine for radical cure of malaria in Irian Jaya, Indonesia. *Annals of Tropical Medicine and Parasitology,* 1997, 91:7–16.

75. Valibayov A et al. Clinical efficacy of chloroquine followed by primaquine for *Plasmodium vivax* treatment in Azerbaijan. *Acta Tropica,* 2003, 88:99–102.

76. Wilairatana P et al. Efficacy of primaquine regimens for primaquine-resistant *Plasmodium vivax* malaria in Thailand. *American Journal of Tropical Medicine and Hygiene,* 1999, 61:973–977.

77. Baird JK et al. Diagnosis of resistance to chloroquine by *Plasmodium vivax:* timing of recurrence and whole blood chloroquine levels. *American Journal of Tropical Medicine and Hygiene,* 1997, 56: 621–626.

78. Most H et al. Chloroquine for treatment of acute attacks of vivax malaria. *Journal of the American Medical Association,* 1946, 131:963–967.

79. Rowland M, Durani N. Randomized controlled trials of 5- and 14 days primaquine therapy against relapses of vivax malaria in an Afghan refugee settlement in Pakistan. *Transactions of the Royal Society of Tropical Medicine and Hygiene,* 1999, 93:641–643.

80. Dua VK, Sharma VP. *Plasmodium vivax* relapses after 5 days of primaquine treatment, in some industrial complexes of India. *Annals of Tropical Medicine and Parasitology,* 2001, 95:655–659.

81. Adak T, Sharma VP, Orlov VS. Studies on the *Plasmodium vivax* relapse pattern in Delhi, India. *American Journal of Tropical Medicine and Hygiene,* 1998, 59:175–179.

82. Kitchener SJ, Auliff AM, Rieckmann KH. Malaria in the Australian Defense Force during and after participation in the International Force in East Timor (INTERFET). *Medical Journal of Australia,* 2000, 173:583–585.

83. Duarte EC et al. Association of subtherapeutic dosages of a standard drug regimen with failures in preventing relapses of vivax malaria. *American Journal of Tropical Medicine and Hygiene,* 2001, 65:471–476.

84. Durante ME et al. Case report: An unusual late relapse of *Plasmodium vivax* malaria. *American Journal of Tropical Medicine and Hygiene,* 2003, 68:159–160.

85. Pukrittayakamee S et al. Therapeutic responses to antimalarial and antibacterial drugs in vivax malaria. *Acta Tropica,* 2004, 89:351–356.

86. White NJ. The assessment of antimalarial drug efficacy. *Trends in Parasitology,* 2002, 18:458–464.

87. Congpuong K et al. Sensitivity of *Plasmodium vivax* to chloroquine in Sa Kaeo Province, Thailand. *Acta Tropica,* 2002, 83:117–121.

88. Baird JK, Hoffman SL. Primaquine therapy for malaria. *Clinical Infectious Diseases,* 2004, 39:1336–1345.

89. Taylor WR. Antimalarial drug toxicity: a review. *Drug Safety,* 2004, 27:25–61.

90. Leslie T et al. Compliance with 14-day primaquine therapy for radical cure of vivax malaria – a randomized placebo-controlled trial comparing unsupervised with supervised treatment. *Transactions of the Royal Society of Tropical Medicine and Hygiene,* 2004, 98:168–173.

91. Walsh DS et al. Efficacy of monthly tafenoquine for prophylaxis of *Plasmodium vivax* and multidrug-resistant *P. falciparum* malaria. *Journal of Infectious Diseases,* 2004, 190:1456–1463.

92. Chotivanich K et al. Ex-vivo short-term culture and developmental assessment of *Plasmodium vivax*. *Transactions of the Royal Society of Tropical Medicine and Hygiene,* 2001, 95:677–680.

93. Tasanor O et al. An *in vitro* system for assessing the sensitivity of *Plasmodium vivax* to chloroquine. *Acta Tropica,* 2002, 83:49–61.

94. Russell BM et al. Simple *in vitro* assay for determining the sensitivity of *Plasmodium vivax* isolates from fresh human blood to antimalarials in areas where *P. vivax* is endemic. *Antimicrobial Agents and Chemotherapy,* 2003, 47:170–173.

95. *Assessment and monitoring of antimalarial drug efficacy for the treatment of uncomplicated falciparum malaria.* Geneva, World Health Organization, 2003.

A